FLASHING LIGHTS AT NIGHT

The Miraculous Story of a Child's Recovery from a Traumatic Brain Injury

A TRUE STORY

BY

ANN McRAE

Also by ANN McRAE

Love, Life, Loss and Other Four-Letter Words:
Messages to Kathie (2020).
Alia's Voice: A Syrian Refugee in Canada (2023)
Mousa From Nowhere (2025)

FLASHING LIGHTS AT NIGHT

The Miraculous Recovery of a Child
from a Serious Brain Injury

A TRUE STORY

BY

ANN McRAE

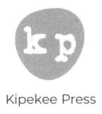

Kipekee Press

ISBN paperback: 978-1-990728-49-5
ISBN hardcover: 978-1-990728-50-1
ISBN eBook: 978-1-990728-56-3
ISBN audiobook: 978-1-990728-53-2

PUBLISHED BY KIPEKEE PRESS in Hamilton, Ontario, Canada.

DEDICATION

This book is dedicated to first responders, health care professionals, and trauma counsellors.

Thank you.

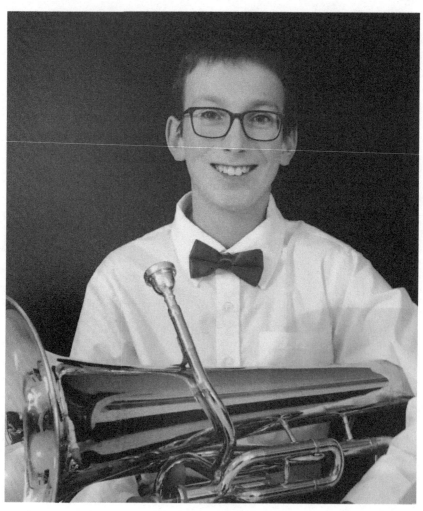

1 Caleb Pate, eleven years old.

TABLE OF CONTENTS

MAP:
CALEB'S VIEW OF NORTH BRANTFORD

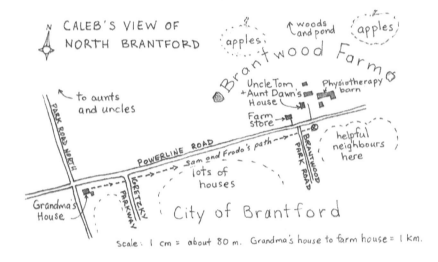

CALEB'S VIEW OF NORTH BRANTFORD

Scale: 1 cm = about 80 m. Grandma's house to farm house = 1 km.

CHARACTERS APPEARING IN THIS TRUE STORY

Caleb Pate, eleven years old in 2022, lives at Gloryview Farm, Stewart Valley, Saskatchewan.

Bruce and Bettina Pate, Caleb's parents.

Bruce and Bettina's younger children: **Eliza, Ethan and Lukas.**

Micah Bruinsma (Bettina's older son and Bruce's stepson), lives in Swift Current, Saskatchewan.

Doreen Pate, Bruce's mother

Tom and Dawn Pate, proprietors of Brantwood Farm on Powerline Road, Bruce's brother and his sister-in-law.

Kara Pate, farm store manager, daughter of Tom and Dawn.

Erica Pate, employed at the Ontario Ministry of Agriculture and Food, daughter of Tom and Dawn

Andrew Pate, field crops manager, son of Tom and Dawn.

Bruce's other siblings: **Wilson Pate, Jim Pate, John Pate;**

Manfred and Renate Kurshner, Bettina Pate's parents, living at Gloryview Farm, Stewart Valley, Saskatchewan, where Bruce and Bettina's family also lives.

Other family members: Aunt Ann Wilson; Aunt Heather Pate, married to Jim Pate; cousin, Ann (the author) and her husband, the Rev. Jim Cairney.

Medical characters:

Dr. Ajani, pediatric neurosurgeon, McMaster Children's Hospital, Hamilton.

Brooke Newsome (now Brooke Pate), pediatric emergency nurse, McMaster Children's Hospital, fiancé of Andrew Pate, at the time of writing.

A host of doctors, residents, occupational and physical therapists, counsellors at McMaster Children's Hospital in Hamilton and at Holland Bloorview Kids Rehabilitation Hospital in Toronto.

PROLOGUE

Your brain has three parts: there is a generator, wiring, and the
light bulbs at the ends of the wiring.

—Dr. Olufemi Ajani,
Pediatric Neurosurgeon, Hamilton, Ontario.

Caleb Pate's lights went out on December 22, 2022 at 5:15 p.m. He was eleven years old. His had been an active and happy life. Was it suddenly over?

His admission notes at McMaster Children's Hospital tell a bleak story. "Brain trauma" is the chilling phrase used in the medical world for his type of head injury. It is measured using the Glasgow Coma Score or GCS. Scores in this scale range from three to fifteen, where numbers lower than five suggest an 80% chance of being in a lasting vegetative state, or worse. Caleb's GCS score on the dark night of December 22 was six.

SECTION ONE

SUNSET

CHAPTER ONE

~~~~~

DECEMBER 22, 2022, 5:05 PM - CHRISTMAS AT GRANDMA'S

Spending the Christmas break with Bruce's family in Brantford, Ontario, was both a tradition and a treat for Bruce and Bettina and their young family. The four children looked forward to presents, of course, but they also looked forward to hugs from Grandma and visiting their aunts and uncles, and there would be plenty of opportunities to play with their many cousins. Bruce and Bettina brought Caleb, eleven, Eliza, nine, and the little ones, four-year-old Ethan and three-year-old Lukas on the trek from Stewart Valley, Saskatchewan, to Ontario every year just before Christmas. Bettina's oldest boy, Micah, Bruce's stepson, was working in Swift Current, where he lived, and was unable to join them.

As usual, their travel day on Wednesday was a bit of an ordeal: coping with baggage, presents, snowsuits, children in airports. It was past midnight, early Thursday morning, when they finally arrived at Grandma Doreen's house, a white frame house at the corner of Park and Powerline Road. It had long been known as "Grandma's house;" even before Grandma Doreen, it had been occupied by Bruce's grandmother. In those early days, the entire family operation, Brantwood Farm, was on one large property on the south side of Powerline. Over a period of seventy years, the city boundary steadily encroached from the south, bringing streets, houses, and stoplights.

Now the primary site of Brantwood Farm is on the opposite side of the road from Grandma's House. The farm produce store, facing the road, is near the home built by Tom and Dawn. A grove of maple and fir trees screens the new Brantwood farmhouse from the road, together with its cluster of barns, drive sheds and a greenhouse. Of the former farm called Brantwood, on the South side of Powerline, only Grandma's house remains, surrounded by housing developments. Over those years, the original narrow, gravel track that was Powerline Road has become a paved, well-travelled, suburban artery.

Far from the road, at the new Brantwood, a paradise for children has been created in a forest, well beyond the farm buildings, the apple orchards and the pumpkin fields; a paradise long enjoyed by many Brantford families. A cable-bridge spans the muddy brook. Paths wind around the not-yet-frozen skating pond and through the woods to a multi-level play fort with slides and climbing apparatus, where young imaginations could spread their wings.

Tired from the trip but excited to be at Grandma's, the children straggled to the kitchen for a late breakfast, and then were eager to pile into Bruce's borrowed van to be dropped off at Tom and Dawn's house. After a brief greeting to their aunt and uncle, four children prepared to romp down the lane, heading for the skating pond trails at the farthest end of the farm. Bruce caught Caleb's attention just before they all bolted, reminding him that the afternoon would be interrupted by a trip to a mall in Brantford so that Caleb could find a Christmas present for Grandma. Caleb rolled his eyes but nodded. At the idea of going to a mall, a rare event for a country boy, Ethan piped up, "Can I come too, Dad?"

"Sure, why not?" replied Bruce. He smiled at the adults, shrugging at the banging of doors as the children raced out. Dawn's offer of coffee was warmly received by he and Bettina, who were both feeling the effects of time zones and a short night.

In midafternoon, Bruce and Bettina drove the van to the back of Tom's farm to round up the kids, who were tired and slightly muddy after their adventures. Bruce dropped Bettina, Eliza and Lukas at Grandma's house to have a snack and get cleaned up for supper, while he drove Caleb and Ethan to Brantford to join the throngs of last-minute shoppers. Eliza and Lukas settled in to make some Christmas decorations with paper and markers in Grandma's kitchen.

At around 5:30, Bruce expected to be back to take his family and his mother to Tom and Dawn's home for supper. Bettina kept her eye on the clock, planning to set out on the twelve-minute walk to Brant-wood with Eliza and Lukas, perhaps arriving in time to help Dawn with last-minute preparations.

Bruce's brother, Tom Pate, and his wife Dawn and their family had operated the Powerline Road location of Brantwood Farm for thirty years, making it into a family activity centre with festivals for every season: pick-your-own strawberries, flowers, apples and pumpkins. Tom and Dawn had recently stepped back from management, handing the reins to their daughter Kara and son Andrew, Bruce's niece and nephew.

As the evening shadows lengthened, Bettina called to Eliza and Lukas to tidy up and get their coats. She hoped the walk would help three-year-old Lukas burn off some energy before dinner.

Bettina was about to step outside with Eliza and Lukas when they heard the gravel crunching as Bruce's van rolled to a stop outside the house. Caleb bounded out of the van, ready to join the walking group, calling out to Eliza as he slipped into character for their favourite game of adventure. Bruce helped Ethan climb out of the van, then gathered up the parcels they had purchased.

"We gotta hurry, Sam, before the Ring Wraiths catch up to us." He was always Frodo to her Sam when they played at *Lord of the Rings*. In response, Eliza instantly became Sam, the faithful companion. She set her face in a grim frown and pretended to rein in an impatient steed that she was riding in her imagination.

Bettina held up her hand in a gesture that slowed Caleb down, shook her head at him, and was staring at a patch of dirt on the legs of his jeans as she spoke: "Not so fast, there, Caleb. What's this? Looks like dried mud splashes."

"It was muddy back at the pond this afternoon," Caleb offered with a shrug, seeming surprised to see several smears on both of his pant-legs. His attempt to brush them off only smudged the denim.

"Sorry, buddy, but you can't show up at the church to sing carols after supper in muddy jeans. Run inside and find something else. We'll wait."

Bruce, who had been opening the door for Ethan on his way into the house, now held the door open for Caleb with a nod toward the house and a look that said, "You heard your mother." Caleb spun around, bounded up four steps and disappeared into Grandma's house. Bruce and Ethan followed. Little blond Ethan was too tired to join the walkers and was looking forward to a bit of story time with Grandma.

As Bettina waited outside with Eliza and Lukas, she realized that Eliza and Caleb would scamper off like wild rabbits, playing their game and arriving at Tom and Dawn's long before she and Lukas got there. She felt sorry for Lukas, as instead of the fun walk with Eliza that he may be envisioning, he would have to spend the long walk in the almost-dark with just Mom. She knew he loved his time with her, but even so, she also knew it would not be as much fun for him as walking with his big sister.

Caleb burst through the door moments later, in his new black jeans. He tugged his Calgary Flames toque down over tousled brown hair and straightened his red-framed glasses. He wore his black school-band sweater under an unzipped winter jacket, and, as Bettina noticed, there was no sign of gloves. As he thundered down the four wooden steps, his hazel eyes twinkled, and he slipped back into character as Frodo. He called out to Eliza, "C'mon, Sam! Let's go!" His role was always the adventurous hero. Eliza, as little sister, had to be content to follow where he led. With a whoop, they were off at a gallop on imaginary horses.

The older ones tore off down the grassy verge on the south side of Powerline Road, towards their uncle and aunt's home. The entire family walked this familiar route many times, each time they visited at Grandma's house. The path soon joined a paved walkway under the hydro towers. They would pass the Brantwood Farm store and the intersection of Brantwood Park Drive before finally reaching the rural mailbox that marked Tom and Dawn's lane. Then they could cross over Powerline Road and walk north, along Tom and Dawn's maple-shaded lane.

After the others set off, Grandma took little Ethan to read picture books on the sofa with her, giving Bruce a few minutes to step into the shower. Soon they would be due at his eldest brother's house for dinner and, as Bruce and Bettina had been up early that morning with the kids, and busy all day, a hot shower was a most welcome bit of down-time. Bruce smiled, knowing that his children had inevitably found the muddiest spots during their day of play, just as he himself had during his childhood. Bruce heard the kitchen door slam as Caleb sprinted out to join the others outside. He could hear his four-year-old discussing with Grandma which picture book he would like her to read to him. Then Bruce turned the shower on. Under the rushing water, he didn't hear anything else for several minutes.

Ah, peace.

CHAPTER TWO

5: 10 PM, GRANDMA'S HOUSE

On December 22, 2022, the sun set at 4:49 p.m. By 5: 15, the only light in the sky was a band of pale yellow just above the western horizon. Grandma's living room had windows facing west where black silhouettes of bare trees formed a filigree pattern, overlaying the outlines of a neighbour's farm buildings.

Doreen Pate was ninety-two and slowing down. For decades she was actively involved in apple sales at the farm store, watching it grow to a multi-faceted business. Although she was having a little trouble with her vision, Grandma Pate was able to read storybooks with Ethan, her four-year-old grandson. Bruce was still in the shower when they finished the first book, so she asked Ethan to pick another from her shelf.

Powerline gets its less-than-scenic name from a long row of tall steel structures carrying hydro cables high above the ground. The towers, like an endless column of mechanical soldiers, carry electricity from Niagara, through Burlington, to points west of Brantford. The towers have been marching in place for so long that the road's name before 1915 is lost in the mists of time. Farms along this road were among the first to be "electrified" in the previous century.

Doreen heard Bruce's phone buzzing faintly somewhere while he was showering, and ignored it, turning her complete attention to the child snuggled up to her. Ethan leaned in as she read. With three siblings at home, he rarely got to choose the book. Even more wonderful was they could go at his pace and that he got to turn the pages. His day was almost perfect.

Ethan's day got even better when they heard sirens coming close. Such a thing never happened at home in rural Saskatchewan. Grandma said, "Look Ethan, it's a fire truck, I think. Yes! A small one. And it's going to turn and go past us!"

The sirens got very loud as the Emergency Services van slowed down to make the turn at the intersection of Park Road and Powerline. Being on a corner lot, Grandma's house had excellent views of both roads, and Ethan took full advantage. He put his hands over his ears, but eagerly moved to the window, watching the flashing lights glittering in the twilight.

When the emergency vehicle had disappeared from view, they returned to the sofa. Doreen, with Ethan's insistent help, found the page and resumed reading aloud. After a few short moments, they heard another siren. It, too, seemed to be coming very close. Hopeful of seeing yet another emergency vehicle, Ethan hopped up from the sofa and headed for the living room window. Two in one day!

Visits to Grandma's house were always good, but this was exceptional. Sure enough, another set of flashing lights rounded the corner. This time, it was not like the first truck. It was a white ambulance! The siren was different from the fire vehicle. Ethan hoped Grandma would take him outside so they could watch it disappear down the road, but she thought it would be better to keep reading. So they did.

They had read only two pages of their second book when a third siren drew Ethan back to the window. Wow! Another set of flashing lights sent red and blue spears of light scattering throughout Doreen's living and dining room, bouncing off every glass or polished surface in her home.

"Amb-bin-ants!" Ethan announced, thrilled to now be an expert in such matters. The second white cube van rounded the corner and screamed down Powerline Road.

"Well, well. Three ambulances or fire trucks. My goodness, Ethan—that must have been a pretty big accident!"

Doreen noticed the floor creaking overhead. Bruce, evidently finished his shower, was moving around in the bedroom, suddenly making a lot of noise. They would be leaving for dinner as soon as Bruce was dressed. Doreen was ready, as was Ethan. She thumbed the picture book: six pages left. Little Ethan wasn't going to find out how the book ended unless they pressed on. They prepared to resume reading. This time, Doreen let Ethan find the page where they had left off.

Bruce came down the stairs at a trot, still buttoning his shirt.

"Mom, get your coat. We're going. I got a phone message from Dawn. Caleb's been in an accident. I have to find Bettina's bag and take her wallet to her. Let's go, Ethan, right away! Get your coat on!"

Short minutes later, Ethan, Bruce, and Doreen were bundled in their winter coats and in Bruce's van. The drive to Tom's would take just over a minute, assuming he hit the first traffic light when it was green. It was.

Bruce's van was closing in on the cluster of emergency vehicles. Faces were pressed to the windows in several of the houses on the south side of Powerline Road. Pulsing blue and red lights and vehicles parked at angles across the now-dark road contributed to a sense of general chaos, but Bruce stayed calm. It seemed more sensible to park at the farm store, so he wheeled left before he reached the emergency vehicles into the dark parking lot.

The store had closed at five and the lot was empty. Leaving his van running to keep Doreen and Ethan warm, he grabbed Bettina's wallet. As Bruce loped across the road, he could see a stretcher being rolled toward the back of one of the ambulances. There was a body on it.

CHAPTER THREE

〜

5:15 PM, ELIZA

Initially, the scene was in twilight, dimly lit from streetlamps at the nearby intersection of Powerline Road with Brantwood Park Drive. The taillights of the car that had braked and swerved, in an attempt to miss Caleb, added an eerie reddish glow. On Powerline Road, the driver had seen only a shadow suddenly emerging from the right, and a dark figure was caught in his headlight beams. Before abruptly braking and swerving, he had no time to assess whether it was human or animal, adult or child. The sickening thump was almost simultaneous with jamming his foot on the brake. The driver's evasive action may have saved Caleb from a much worse outcome.

Caleb had his back to the approaching car. Eliza, nine years old, was mere centimetres from Caleb when the side of the car, near the front wheel, struck a glancing blow at about hip level. His slim upper body and back made contact with the windshield. The back of Caleb's head struck the top of the windshield, while the car's side-mirror scooped him off the ground. As the mirror broke off under the force of the impact, Caleb slid off the car and landed almost flat, skidding along the pavement on his back.

Eliza saw her brother hit the ground and reacted immediately. She felt he was in danger while lying on the pavement, on his back, possibly in the path of other cars, and in the dark. He did not appear to be doing

self, and actually not moving at all. Calling his
, and getting no response, she grabbed him under
auled with all her strength. She dug in with her heels
id kept dragging until he was lying on the safer, grassy
ids were fluttering, but otherwise he was not moving. He
w.   ot answering her. Not even "Thanks" or "I'm okay." It was
clear ι her that something was seriously wrong.

A car door opened in the darkness, a short distance away. She did not take her eyes off Caleb, but she could tell that the driver had stopped his vehicle and emerged. His first words sounded angry.

"Dude, what were you doing? Where did you come from? You ran right into me."

Eliza was stunned that the driver seemed to be speaking to Caleb, and to be unaware that Caleb was injured.

The appearance of two children may have surprised the driver even more than the impact of a body on his car. When the driver got closer to Eliza, he realized how young both children were. "Hey, kid, do you live around here? Can you go get someone?"

Eliza kept her attention focused on Caleb. She did not look up.

"Do you live near here?" he repeated.

Eliza felt frozen. She wasn't sure she wanted to leave Caleb alone with just this stranger, the driver, who seemed a bit angry.

She had just located her brother's glasses, lying broken on the pavement. She carefully placed the broken glasses near his head. Everything was a turmoil in her mind. How far behind them was their mom? When would she catch up? Who could she trust?

The driver was no longer trying to get Eliza to speak to him. She thought maybe he was on his phone, but she didn't want to look up. She continued to ignore him and focus on her brother. What should she do for Caleb until her mom got there? There must be something, she thought. She took off her coat and laid it over him for extra warmth.

People were emerging from their houses on the south side of Powerline Road. At least one person had seen or heard the accident through a kitchen window. Quickly, neighbours alerted each other. A man came out of his yard and crossed in the twilight to where Caleb was lying. He reached Eliza's side shortly after the driver. Seeing that she was a young child, he asked the same question the driver had just posed, "Do you live nearby? Can you go and get anyone?"

Eliza nodded. She pointed to the house; its lights were barely visible through a stand of trees on the north side of the road. "That's my Aunt Dawn and Uncle Tom's. We were going there for dinner..." Their lane was directly opposite the spot where Caleb was lying. A yard light illuminated part of the lane near the house. The man knelt down beside Eliza and encouraged her: "You go. I'll stay with him."

Eliza was uncertain about taking direction from strangers, and doubtful about whether she should leave Caleb's side before her mother got there. She could not tear her gaze from Caleb's face, immobile except for the tremor in his eyelids.

By now, more cars were stopping and more people were coming out of houses. A woman from a nearby house arrived and quickly knelt on the other side of Caleb. She put her hand beside his neck. Eliza knew she was checking for a pulse. Without taking her eyes off Caleb, the woman called out to the gathering crowd, "Has anyone called an ambulance?"

"Yes. On its way," came a reply from a man's voice in the darkness.

The woman's calm manner was very reassuring to Eliza. She now felt there were enough adults around that it was safe to leave Caleb in their care, and not to wait any longer for her mother. Tears were stinging in her eyes. She didn't want to cry with all these strangers around.

Sensing her uncertainty, the man said, again, "Go. Get your aunt or uncle. We'll take care of him." The woman nodded to her in agreement and patted her hand.

Eliza jumped to her feet, eager to have something useful to do. Checking the road carefully this time, Eliza took off at a run toward Tom and Dawn's house.

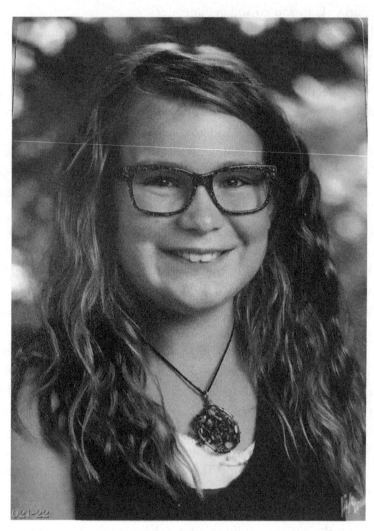

Eliza Pate, nine years old.

CHAPTER FOUR

5:17 PM, DAWN'S KITCHEN

"**A**unt Dawn, Caleb's been hit by a car and his glasses are broken." From the kitchen, Dawn Pate heard her front door open, and then the sobbing, gasping voice of her nine-year-old niece. All Dawn heard was "… his glasses are broken." At first Dawn didn't absorb what Eliza had said, but it was apparently about Caleb. Dawn asked, "Where is Caleb?"

Eliza stood sobbing in the front hall, still holding the handle of the open door. Dawn went to her, hugged the tall girl to calm her down, and gently closed the door. She saw that, although Eliza had winter boots on, she was wearing only a thin sweater over her jeans. Catching her breath, Eliza spoke again between sobs, "Caleb was hit by a car."

"Where? Where is Caleb?"

"Near the road. I pulled him off. We were just coming here. Mom and Lukas were behind us."

Dawn had been preparing dinner, having already set the table for nine: Bruce and Bettina's family and her mother-in-law, Doreen, Tom, and herself. She was putting dinner in the oven just as Eliza appeared.

Sliding her family's dinner into the oven, she threw off her apron and grabbed her coat and cellphone. She jammed her feet into a pair of boots. For Eliza, Dawn grabbed another coat from the pegs near the door—one of her own, but better than nothing for the child.

"Take me to him."

Eliza was already out the door ahead of her.

The lane was shadowy, overhung with trees. The only light was behind them. Dawn began dialing 911 with fumbling fingers as she and Eliza hurried along in semi-darkness. In less than a minute, they reached the road, just as Dawn connected with a 911 dispatcher. The operator was already aware of the accident and assured Dawn that first responders were on the way. However, the first caller had not been able to give any details about the name or age of the injured person, or the exact location. Dawn and Eliza paused at the end of the lane before crossing the road, while Dawn answered the dispatcher's questions. Sirens could be heard in the distance.

Although night was falling rapidly, Dawn could see a woman kneeling beside the figure of Caleb stretched out on the grass. Someone had covered Caleb up to his chin with a blanket. The woman at his side did not appear to be her sister-in-law, Bettina. Where was Bettina?

CHAPTER FIVE

~~~~~

5:05 PM MOM!

Lukas had been looking forward to walking with Mom and 'Liza. Watching his big brother and sister run far ahead of them toward Uncle Tom's meant he was going to walk with just Mom. The blond-haired three-year-old Lukas enjoyed his time with Mom, but he was wistful, watching his older siblings disappear into the gloom. They were close friends, Eliza and Caleb, and had games they did not share with him and Ethan.

The older children would cover the path to Tom and Dawn's in seven or eight minutes, maybe less, pausing only at two intersections along the way, to catch their breath. For Bettina and Lukas, it would take almost three times as long.

"Can Dad and Ethan walk with us, Mom?"

"No, Lukie. They'll come with Grandma. You can walk with me. You're a big boy, Lukie." Slightly mollified to know that Mom considered him a "big boy", Lukas took her hand, and they set off.

Bettina's stroll along the bike path, parallel to Powerline Road, was as relaxed as it could be, except for shortening her stride so that Lukas could keep up. There was no snow; the paved path was dry.

At first, Bettina was able to interest Lukas in the construction site that wrapped around the back of Grandma's house and yard. It was more spooky than interesting in the waning light.

They crossed under the steely-grey wash of artificial light from the buzzing overhead lamps at Gretzky Parkway after waiting for the "walk" signal. They came to an established neighbourhood. Lights from the houses were screened by a row of solid board fences. Dogs barked at them from the enclosed yards. The path, under the hydro towers, was paved for about half a kilometer.

Ahead of her, Bettina could no longer see Eliza and Caleb in the gathering darkness. There were streetlights at the intersection of Powerline and Gretzky Parkway, a road named after local hockey hero, Wayne Gretzky. After those lights, there was nothing until the smaller intersection of Brantwood Park Drive, about a half-kilometer away.

Bettina hoped the older children would offer to help Aunt Dawn when they arrived, long before she, Bruce, Grandma, and the little boys got there. Then Bettina sighed: no, the draw of the games and toys in Dawn's basement would be irresistible. Let kids be kids.

In the distance, Bettina saw a confusion of people coming out of the houses on the south side of Powerline, returning through the garden gates, then re-emerging. A small group was forming on the same side of the road she was following with Lukas. Maybe a pizza delivery driver had stopped on Powerline, and a customer was coming out to meet the driver? Or maybe not. There were too many people for that to make sense.

Lukas was talking to her, but Bettina didn't hear him. Her instincts were focused on the dimly lit scene far ahead of her, where something was not right. She was still four or five minutes away from what might have been a car accident, but she saw only one car. Another vehicle had stopped, but it was on the other side, going the opposite way. That made little sense. What was going on up there?

She pulled a little harder on Lukas, and encouraged him to trot along a little faster, so they could find out what was happening near Aunt Dawn and Uncle Tom's place. As they got closer, they passed through a pool of pale light as they crossed the intersection with Brantwood Park Drive. Then it was dark again as they approached Tom and

Dawn's mailbox. Finally Bettina was able to pick out details: some-thing, or someone, was lying in the grass.

A small knot of people was standing or crouching in the same area. She didn't see Eliza or Caleb among them, which gave her a rush of relief; it didn't last long.

Two more figures were crossing from the north side of Powerline. When they crossed into the headlight beams from the parked car, she saw them in silhouette: her sister-in-law Dawn with Eliza. Still puzzled, Bettina quickened her pace to a brisk walk, almost towing Lukas, who was now curious and doing his best to keep up.

Bettina was now close enough for Eliza to see her. A siren in the distance, and the murmur of voices drowned out Eliza's, but Bettina could see the word "Mom!" on her lips, and then saw Eliza form another word that must have been "Caleb." Bettina gasped. She and Lukas ran toward the group of people.

Bettina prayed for calm as she pounded along the path. "Peace, not panic, Lord," she breathed. She was now beyond the end of the paved path, on bare dry ground, worn by many feet and bicycles. Lukas' little legs were churning along beside her.

Eliza called out to her again, and this time, Bettina was near enough to hear clearly:

"Mom! Caleb was hit by a car and his glasses are broken." Some of this information seemed so trivial to Bettina that it was hard to take Eliza seriously. Bettina's first reaction was to say to Eliza, "Are you kidding me?"

In the next stride, Bettina released Lukas' hand, reached Caleb, and crouched beside his motionless form, seeing for herself that Eliza was serious.

A stranger was already kneeling at Caleb's side when Bettina arrived. The woman turned and said to Bettina in a calm, confident voice, "He's breathing and his pulse is strong."

These words shocked Bettina into automatically performing the check that she, as a nurse, had performed on hundreds of emergency-room patients. She observed the regular rising and falling of her son's chest, while reaching to take his pulse and mentally counting to judge his heart rate. Her hand was trembling in a way that she had never experienced when measuring a patient's pulse. She called his name over and over, hoping his eyes would open at the sound of her voice. Nothing. After several tries, she recognized that he could not respond.

Bettina then turned to the woman who was still kneeling beside her, whose calm assurance had been just what Bettina needed. "Thank you so much for being here with him," she whispered, still slightly breathless from her run.

"I'm a nurse," came the woman's whispered answer.

"So am I," was Bettina's response. It was an instant bond for them.

"Has anyone called for an ambulance?" Bettina called out.

"Yes," the man in the darkness repeated. Almost at the same time, Dawn added, "I just called 911. The dispatcher said they had already received a request for an ambulance. I think I can see it at the corner."

After crossing the road with Dawn, Eliza had come to Bettina's side, and had taken Lukas' hand. He had come to a halt behind Bettina, mute, confused and transfixed by the scene before him. He grabbed Eliza's hand and held it to his face with both of his, while continuing to stare, wide-eyed. Eliza looked gratefully at the woman who had reassured her mom, then looked at Caleb again, and was startled.

"Hey, where's my jacket? I left it over him. It's gone."

"It's underneath him," said the woman, lifting the blanket so that Eliza could see her jacket under his head and shoulders. Dawn walked around Caleb, gathered up Eliza and Lukas, and wondered if she should stay or get the children to her warm house.

Time seemed to slow to a stop while they waited for the emergency services to arrive. Bettina, kneeling near Caleb's head, reached out to place a hand out to Caleb's forehead as she prayed for him. The act of praying spread a feeling of peace over her whole body, which had been pumping adrenalin and making her heart thump so hard that she imagined she could hear the pounding in her ears. Very slowly and deliberately, she took a deep breath and let it out gradually. She calmly thought, "Caleb needs me to be here, to be strong. I can do this for him. Thank you, God, for strength."

Seeing Caleb's toque and broken glasses neatly placed on the grass by his head, Bettina calmly slipped them into her coat pocket. Astonishingly, the lenses were lightly scuffed but intact. Only an arm of the glasses had broken.

The screaming sirens of an emergency services vehicle blotted out all thought and conversation for a few seconds, then mercifully went silent as the vehicle rolled in and parked on the shoulder of the road. Its headlights raked over the grassy roadside, but failed to cast much light on Caleb. Flashing lights pulsated red and blue on the faces of those gathered.

While the driver was still positioning the vehicle, a lanky young man with short red hair bolted from the passenger seat and knelt in the grass beside Bettina. He introduced himself as a paramedic. He spoke to her as he scanned Caleb for signs of injuries. The angled headlight beams from the emergency vehicle were all wrong. The paramedic shouted to his partner or anyone who could hear, "I need a light! I can't see."

Bettina pulled her cell phone out of a pocket and focused its flashlight on Caleb. The paramedic confirmed what the first woman had said to Bettina: Caleb was breathing and had a strong pulse. He was unable to identify any injuries, as there was no sign of blood on Caleb's clothing.

Bettina was still holding her phone-flashlight aimed at Caleb when she noticed the phone in Dawn's hand. "Dawn," she called to get her attention, "Please call Bruce, tell him to get here right away. Tell him to bring my wallet."

Another siren heralded a second vehicle, an ambulance. It parked on the road, very close to where Caleb was lying, leaving its flashing lights on but turning off the siren. Within seconds a police cruiser, also lit up with flashers, approached from the opposite direction. The officer angled it across Powerline Road to deter anyone thinking of using the road. Then, once parked, the officer leapt out and ran over to confer with the paramedics, who were now both kneeling in the grass assessing Caleb. Crouching, the officer nodded a greeting to them, and asked, "How is he?"

The red-haired paramedic confirmed to the police officer the information that the woman had given Bettina: Caleb's pulse was strong, and he was breathing. He turned to his colleague.

"We're going to add a mask anyway," he advised, and she nodded. This second paramedic, a blond woman with her hair tied in a ponytail, had just pulled an oxygen mask out of their equipment bag.

A short distance away from them, the ambulance doors opened, spilling a little more light on the grassy area. Two more paramedics unloaded a stretcher, all the while speaking with the first two, to gather information about Caleb.

Bettina was an experienced emergency-room nurse, but this crisis found her outside her normal hospital environment. It was reassuring to see the team of first responders efficiently assessing and preparing Caleb to be loaded onto the stretcher. Usually she dealt with patients and families after the ambulance ride.

She overheard the medics briefing the hospital's emergency staff, in a staccato conversation filled with numbers and facts. She had been at the receiving end of such calls dozens of times, while on duty in the emergency room where she worked. She felt detached from reality, watching "her work" being done here in the chilly darkness by others. Then she snapped back to the moment, as one of the paramedics had approached her, needing information.

More and more flashing lights lit up the night sky as a second ambulance arrived, followed by another police cruiser. Dawn, Eliza and Bettina were kept busy answering the questions fired at them by the ambulance attendants, who were still on the phone with the Emergency Department at McMaster Children's Hospital giving as much information about the incoming patient's condition as they could. The police officer was also standing with his notepad open, collecting contact information from everyone before the ambulance left.

What's his name?... Spell that, please... Where does he live? Sas-katchewan? ... Who is he visiting here?... What's your name?... That's your house right there?... You are Mrs. Pate, then?... Oh, you are all Pates. Ok. Did you see what happened?... Who saw what happened?... How old are you?... You pulled him off the road? By yourself? You're a strong girl. Great job, kid. I'll need to talk to you later, ok?... Who is the mother? Ok, what's your name?... Phone number?... You'll need to go in the ambulance, ma'am. I can talk to you later. ...Who else saw what happened? ...Your name?... and phone number, sir?

The ambulance attendants arranged the collapsed stretcher beside Caleb. Bettina was still holding the light. One spoke to her: "I under-stand you're a nurse, ma'am. That might be useful once we're underway, but don't worry, we've got this. Once we get him loaded, you just hold his hand and talk to him. We'll do the rest. Don't worry. His pulse is good, he's breathing, and he can feel pain, though he doesn't seem to be in any pain, as far as we can tell. We don't need your flashlight any more, thanks. Are you ok, ma'am?"

Bettina slipped her cell phone into her pocket and took a deep breath, before answering. A shudder went through her.

"Yes. Yes, I'm fine... Thank you." Only then did she realize she was trembling.

Dawn Pate was suddenly aware that the brave nine-year-old girl at her side had become very quiet. When she looked down at Eliza's face, Dawn saw the furrowed brow, clenched lips and pale skin. Until now, Eliza had seemed remarkably calm and in control. Dawn thought she must be worried about Caleb, so she tightened her one-arm hug. Lukas was clinging to Dawn's other arm as if glued on. Dawn said quietly in Eliza's ear, but loud enough for Lukas to hear also, "The paramedics are taking good care of him. He'll be at the hospital in just a few minutes."

"The nice lady told me he is not dead," Eliza said in a voice that was on the edge of crying. "It's not that. It's the flashing lights, they're giv-ing me a headache." She covered her eyes with her hands. Dawn pulled her closer and made her stop looking at Caleb.

"We aren't needed here anymore, are we?" Dawn asked the police officer, who paused his notetaking and looked at the children with her: fearful-looking Lukas staring back at him, and Eliza, now crumpled, with her face pressed into Dawn's shoulder.

"No, no, of course not, please take the kids home, Mrs. Pate. I'll come and talk to you later." Dawn led Eliza and Lukas across the road and disappeared into what was now deepening night.

The red-haired fire paramedic conferred with the ambulance team. "I'd like to ride along. I can hold his head until we get to Hamilton," he said. The ambulance crew agreed.

Bettina was alarmed. Hamilton? Wasn't the local Brantford hospital only ten or twelve minutes away? Then she remembered one of the paramedics had mentioned "McMaster," when speaking to the officer. Of course! They were taking Caleb to McMaster Children's Hospital, one of Canada's leading centres for pediatric care, which was about twenty-five minutes away.

The paramedics were wrapping a neck brace around Caleb, in preparation for transferring him to the stretcher. Bettina had wanted to keep one hand on Caleb while they lifted his slight body onto the stretcher, but she stood back while they fastened the straps around him, realizing they needed room to work.

Bettina was vaguely aware that Dawn had gone back to the farmhouse, taking Eliza and Lukas. Just then Bettina heard Bruce's voice, identifying himself to the police officer. He stepped into the small, shadowy crowd of paramedics and police officers at the open ambulance doors, close to where Caleb was lying motionless, on the stretcher. The team had raised the stretcher to waist-height in preparation for wheeling it to the open doors of the ambulance. The paramedics began to roll the stretcher toward the warm light of the open ambulance.

"He's unconscious and unresponsive to me," were Bettina's first words to Bruce. He wrapped her in a brief but fierce hug. "They're taking him to McMaster."

"You go," he said, holding her shoulders and glancing over her shoulder in the direction of the ambulance. "I have to take Mom and Ethan to Tom's first. Here's your wallet. I'll find you at the hospital."

They watched the ambulance crew slide the stretcher into the vehicle, and begin to secure it. Then it was time for Bettina to climb in. The red-haired paramedic had entered first, and was already at Caleb's head, holding both sides of the neck brace a pre-caution against the bumpy shift from the shoulder of the road onto the pavement. The ambulance started up. Meanwhile another paramedic was adjusting Caleb's oxygen mask, another precaution, since he was breathing on his own. She made ready to close the doors, but Bettina stopped her with a gesture.

"Wait, not yet," said Bettina. "Could we pray for him in the ambulance before we go, please? My husband is right outside. Bruce?" The paramedic looked startled by this suggestion. She looked around to see who "Bruce" was. She saw a slim, athletic-looking man leaning into the open ambulance doors. He reached one hand out to clasp Bettina's outstretched hand. With his other hand on Caleb's leg, Bruce said, "Let's pray."

Bruce prayed. His voice was steady and controlled: "Father, thank you for Caleb. Thank you that you are the Great Physician. We ask for your healing touch on Caleb, in Jesus' name. Amen."

He drew back to let the driver close the doors. Bruce felt total peace that things would be okay. Inside the now-rolling ambulance, Bettina felt the same thing.

Flashers and siren were engaged. Gravel flew. They were off. One of Canada's best pediatric care centres was just thirty minutes away. Twenty-five, with lights and siren. They were expected.

Bruce legged it across Powerline Road, which was lit up like a circus midway by all the flashing lights. Farther down the road, in both directions, more cruisers were moving into position to block off parts of Powerline Road so that officers could assess the accident site.

Bruce reached his still-running van in the parking lot of the farm-store. He jumped in and steered it along a dark and bumpy lane that wound around to the back of his brother Tom's house. Grandma and Ethan were eager to hear his report. He addressed Ethan, but took one hand off the steering wheel to briefly pat his mother's arm.

"Caleb hit his head. He's unconscious, but he's going to be okay. I'll be going to the hospital with Mom, but you'll have a nice dinner here, with Aunt Dawn and Uncle Tom." This was a bold projection, but the strong sense of peace that Bruce had felt, at the door of the ambulance, was still with him.

At the house, he followed his mother and Ethan into the large farm kitchen, where he found one of the officers, still gathering information from Dawn and Eliza. Ethan focused on the basement door, waiting for Dawn's signal that it was okay to go and play with the toys. She smiled and nodded at him, and he was off like a sprinter, to play with Lukas.

The officer already knew that Bruce had not witnessed the accident and was a little surprised to see him. "I'll join you at the hospital later, Mr. Pate, but you can get on your way and be with your wife and your boy. Drive carefully, okay?"

Bruce nodded his thanks. He was about to make his apologies to Dawn, but she faced him with glistening eyes, shook her head and gently shoved him back out the door with just one word.

"Go."

Bruce sat in the van, outside the farmhouse, headlights on, motor running. Glancing out from her kitchen, Dawn couldn't understand what she was seeing: why wasn't her brother-in-law on his way to Hamilton, to the hospital? Why was Bruce sitting in his van, apparently doing nothing? Was he looking up the directions to McMaster Hospital? Of course not! It was a straight half-hour drive on Governor's Road—he knew that. He grew up here, after all.

Then she noticed the glow of the cell phone illuminating his face. Later it made sense. He was calling his pastor in Saskatchewan and requesting prayer for Caleb. He also put the word out about the accident to a network of friends in the prairies who, he knew, would pray as soon as they opened his message.

Bruce didn't feel any panic. He felt that God, the God he trusted, was taking care of his family. And that it would be all right. Caleb was beginning a long and difficult journey, for sure, but Bruce had felt that God was in that ambulance, and was watching over his boy. Bruce put the van in gear and launched his own journey toward Hamilton.

SECTION TWO

DARKNESS

CHAPTER SIX

MCMASTER CHILDREN'S HOSPITAL EMERGENCY

Shortly before 6 pm, the ambulance arrived at McMaster Children's Hospital, part of the Hamilton Health Sciences building on the campus of McMaster University. Hamilton is a mid-sized city on the shore of Lake Ontario located a one-hour drive from Toronto, Canada's largest city and just over an hour from the US border.

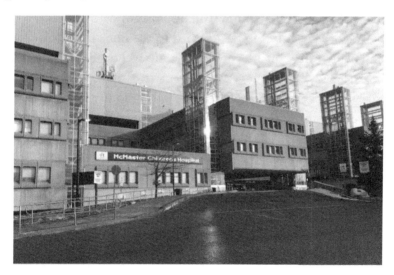

During the ambulance ride, the paramedic holding Caleb's head commented to Bettina that he had played rugby with Andrew Pate and knew the Pate family. His compassionate remarks buoyed Bettina's sense that there was a community of caring all around her.

By the time the ambulance crew unloaded Caleb, his body had assumed a rigid posture described in the medical chart as "decerebrated." He was on his back, neck extended, head tilted back, arms rigid at his side, legs straight with toes pointed down. The first responders recognized this as an indicator of severe brain injury, as did Bettina.

A space in the ER was prepped and ready with both personnel and materials. The ambulance attendants had briefed the Emergency Room team by phone, before the ambulance reached Hamilton.

Brooke Newsome, a young blond nurse, who specialized in Emergency Room care in the pediatric hospital, was on duty and was anticipating the ambulance. She had learned that a new patient would arrive from the Brantford area at around 5:45. The term used to describe the incident was "patient-vehicle trauma."

Brooke's role was to prepare the medications to be hung over the arriving patient's stretcher. She would be ready with the intravenous drugs ready to go, either to be attached to the line already installed by the ambulance crew or inserting a new intravenous line, if more than one was needed. She bent over the new patient and caught a glimpse of his face. He looked familiar, which was jarring to her.

In her nursing experience of just a few years, she had learned that patients will sometimes resemble someone known to, or close to, the health-care worker. Her training was to block out this seeming-familiarity, as it would cause a disruption to the mental focus one needs: any comparisons of the person in distress with the care-givers' own loved ones could cause emotions and sympathy to bubble to the surface. Brooke needed to suppress her emotions, to dissociate herself from the fact that the patient was a child in serious trouble. She was trained to do this, without any emotional moments.

Clothing that impeded any type of treatment was cut away. Intravenous ports already established by the first responders were transferred to the hospital's systems. Sedation was introduced to reduce the patient's natural inclination to thrash their arms and legs. The team needed to be sure his spinal cord had not suffered any damage. The necessity of the oxygen mask was evaluated by the ER team but left in place.

Comatose patients commonly experience nausea and vomiting as they regain consciousness. Because this elevates the risk of asphyxiation, the team intubated Caleb—they inserted a breathing tube through his mouth and down his throat—even though he was breathing without assistance, both in the ambulance and upon arrival.

The team supervisor ordered a chest X-ray and an abdominal ultrasound, to detect any fractures or internal injuries that might not have been noticed by the paramedics. They had observed his movement, although involuntary, of his arms and legs. This made the team was less concerned about damage to his spinal column, yet they sedated him just the same, until tests of his spinal cord could be completed. The observed movement suggested his joints and long bones were intact and that it was unlikely he had fractures or other injuries to his limbs. Treatment of his bruised ankle was less urgent than ascertaining the status of his internal organs.

Brooke knew the ambulance had come from Brantford. A quick glance at the patient's chart provided the young patient's surname: Pate. Brooke had a sudden sinking feeling that this boy was a cousin of Andrew Pate, Brooke's "significant other." Andrew was responsible for field crops and other aspects of his parents' farm on Powerline Road, Brantwood Farm. Brooke would have been at Andrew's parents' home for dinner that night, but getting time off work so close to Christmas was next to impossible, so she had declined the invitation.

Surely this child, who looked like Andrew's cousin from Saskatchewan, wasn't really Caleb? Could Caleb's parents be in Brantford for Christmas? Brooke needed to focus, but had to know. During the admission procedures and tests, a Child Life Worker stood by Caleb's head, explaining each step to him in a quiet, calming voice. Caleb didn't move. His eyes remained closed. It wasn't clear what he could or could not hear.

Brooke moved away from the patient just far enough to scan the people observing through the window to the waiting area. A woman with shoulder-length brown hair and a red Christmas sweatshirt was conferring with ER staff. Could this possibly be Andrew's aunt? She gasped: it was Bettina. Bettina was outside the ER, watching through a window while a social worker and ER doctor were describing everything that was happening to her son. To Caleb.

Brooke looked again at her patient, crushed by the knowledge that he was indeed Caleb, and that his condition was precarious. Brooke knew that she couldn't continue to work on him. She spoke to her charge nurse, who directed another nurse to step in. Brooke left the unit to find a private place to collect herself.

It was nearly six o'clock. Brooke was scheduled to work until eight o'clock, but her charge nurse realized that it wouldn't be realistic to assign Brooke to another patient while a relative of Andrew was receiving critical care. Instead, Brooke was permitted to stay with Bruce and Bettina. There would be a steady flow of reports on Caleb, when his scans started to come back from the diagnostic imaging department. Brooke could help them to understand his condition.

From the moment of his admission, the emergency team wrapped Caleb and his family in a blanket of reassurance. A doctor stood with Bettina outside the room, explaining each step of the first procedures. Brooke knew that although Bettina was also an emergency room nurse, no parents can process all of the medical information about their child in a time of crisis. After taking a few minutes to calm herself, Brooke prepared to go to the waiting area and be there while tests were being done. It would take a few minutes to assess Caleb's condition. She could repeat the information if Bettina wasn't able to focus.

Once it was known that the most serious injury was confined to the brain, treatment measures began. Caleb was prepared for transfer to the Pediatric Intensive Care Unit (PICU), where tests and observations over the succeeding forty hours would determine the extent of the injury to his brain function.

Before transferring him, the emergency room team observed some abrasions on Caleb's right hip and foot, which seemed to confirm that he made contact with the road on his right side. He also had some scrapes on his left shoulder. These injuries were believed to be the site of impact with the car.

Before seven o'clock, Caleb had been moved to a room in the PICU. That was where Brooke found Bettina. By that time, Bruce had arrived, as had John, the Brantford police constable, and a local pastor, Jim, whose wife was Bruce Pate's cousin. Word had spread quickly. They had watched the team prepare Caleb and then wheel him out for a CT scan of his head.

While Brooke was there, Dr. Ajani, a neurosurgeon, brought a report on the first scan of Caleb's head. Although it indicated some bleeding in the brain, this did not seem to concern the neurosurgery team very much. The doctor brought reassurance that although the damage was severe, resulting in unconsciousness, there was reason to hope for a good outcome. It would just take time.

Throughout their time in the waiting area, and later in Caleb's PICU room, Bettina and Bruce were praying that things would go well. They trusted God would take care of their son. Nonetheless, the comfort afforded by the first CT scan was enormous.

Officer John of the Brantford Police Service had come to collect Caleb's clothing, as part of the accident investigation. He lingered at the hospital, out of concern for Caleb's welfare. Noting Bettina's red sweatshirt that said, "Jesus is the reason for the season," John remarked, "I believe that, too, and I'm praying for your son." Bruce and Bettina were very moved by this.

CHAPTER SEVEN

PEDIATRIC INTENSIVE CARE

For all of this time, Caleb was in a cervical collar, and was unconscious— "unresponsive," in the language of the medical records.

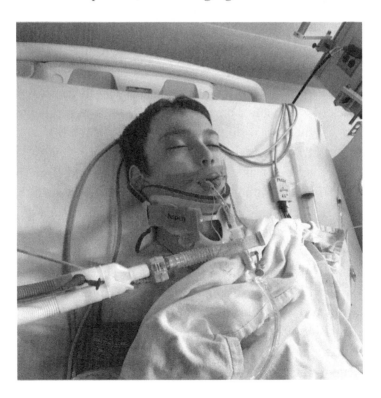

The doctors wanted his sedation to continue, to rest his mind and body overnight. His head was positioned slightly higher than his feet, to reduce swelling in the brain.

The staff team answered as many questions from Bruce and Bettina as they could, but some questions didn't seem to have answers: A surgeon, Dr. Ajani, had boldly forecast "full recovery," but what would that look like, exactly? And how long would it take? What was Caleb experiencing? How could they make it easier for him? Was he experiencing pain? Was the breathing tube necessary? Why was the neck brace left in place?

Amidst all these unknowns, there was a promise that sunshine was on its way. Bruce and Bettina felt a calm, a feeling that things were going to be all right. Prayer and faith held this together; they had confidence in the loving power of God to care for Caleb. Dr. Ajani's comments about "full recovery" stayed with them, although there wasn't much on Caleb's medical charts on which to pin their hopes, so far.

Bettina asked Brooke to go to Tom and Dawn's house, when her shift was over, and help settle the children until Bruce could get there. Bettina would stay in Caleb's room for the night, but Bruce wasn't ready to leave yet. Brooke was the perfect person to take a report on Caleb back to Dawn and Tom's house, which she was pleased to do.

Brooke signed out with her charge nurse, gathered her things and went to her car. Once there, she needed to decompress again, letting herself feel the weight of stress of helping Bettina and Bruce process all the information coming at them. When she could again breathe normally, Brooke called Andrew to report to him first. Then she drove the half-hour to Brantwood. She filled in Doreen, Tom, and Dawn on the optimistic notes in Dr. Ajani's assessment and answered their many questions as best she could. Dawn and Tom had been anxiously watching their phones, but Bettina and Bruce had been too focused to send any news by text, up to that point.

When Brooke arrived at Dawn and Tom's house, Eliza and the boys, Ethan and Lukas, were playing in the basement. After giving the update to the adults, Brooke went downstairs to the playroom. In the cool basement room, she found Ethan and Lukas about to release a couple of toy metal cars on a sloping, curved plastic track. The race course started high at one end of the room and ended with a bold jump onto the carpet. Eliza, still wearing Dawn's jacket open over her jeans and sweater, was acting as chief engineer, stabilizing the track at the higher end, fortifying it using cushions and stuffed animals.

"Hi kids! Wow, have you guys ever grown since last summer! You remember me, right? Brooke?"

She got enthusiastic nods, but it was clearly not a good time to interrupt. Brooke persisted. "Could I at least get 'Merry Christmas, Brooke'?" she prompted, and this time got a chorus of replies.

"That's more like it. I'm sorry to stop the game, but Ethan and Lukas, you are getting a ride to Grandma's house with Aunt Dawn. She's warming up the car. Grandma's getting her coat on. So let's march up those stairs." Seeing Ethan automatically begin picking up cars, she said, "That's okay Ethan, you guys will be back here to continue this race tomorrow. Just leave everything. Gotta get to Grandma's so you can get in your jammies for stories!"

"Jammies?" Ethan burst out with a gleeful guffaw. "Aren't they called p'jamas? And anyway, why are you wearing your p'jamas, Brooke?"

"Jammies, jammies, jammies," teased Brooke, poking his ribs and getting a peal of laughter from Lukas. "Anyway, smart guy, these aren't my pa-ja-mas." She was wearing a matched set of purple scrubs. "This is what nurses wear at my work. Now hustle up those stairs! Eliza, you can stay here for a while longer, okay honey? Don't clean up, it's just fine."

Eliza gratefully collapsed onto the nearby sofa and pushed her horn-rimmed glasses up her nose a bit. Her brown hair was plaited at the back, with some strands escaping and hanging over her face. When the boys had disappeared up the stairs, Brooke cleared a few toys off the sofa and sat beside her.

"I can tell you a bit about Caleb, but I didn't want the little guys to hear." Eliza perked up and smiled at Brooke. "Oh yes, please! Is he awake?"

"No, not yet. He's in a big hospital, the one where I work. You know I'm a nurse, like your mom, right?" Eliza nodded dutifully, but in fact this was news to her. She had never thought of cousin Andrew's girlfriend as having a job. *Did all adults have jobs?* she wondered silently.

"So, I was there when the ambulance came in. I talked to your mom and dad. I heard what a great job you did. He's getting good care—the best there is. It's going to take a while for him to be better, though. Your mom is going to stay with him tonight, but your dad will see you at Grandma's later."

"Will Caleb be awake tomorrow?"

"No, sweetie, probably not. He hit his head pretty hard, so there could be some bleeding inside his head. When that happens, your brain goes to sleep while it tries to fix itself. It's called being in a coma. Have you heard of that?"

Eliza had not. She shook her head, then pondered what Brooke had said.

"I think he was trying to wake up because I saw his eyelids moving a bit. But he couldn't wake up, could he?"

"No, honey, he really couldn't. Do you feel like telling me about what happened?... Only if you want to?"

Eliza turned away from Brooke, imagining the scene.

"We were playing *Lord of the Rings*, like we always do. Caleb was Frodo. He's always Frodo. I'm Sam..." she paused and glanced at Brooke to make sure she was familiar with these characters from J. R. R. Tolkien's book.

"Oh yes, Sam is Frodo's faithful companion, right? Go on."

"...And we had been running away from the Ring Wraiths. We got to the big barrel of gravel that holds up Uncle Tom's mailbox, and we were crouching in the shadows. I was watching the villagers—that's the houses nearby—because Frodo said we couldn't trust them. I was watching through pretend binoculars, like this." She cupped a hand on the sides of her glasses as if scoping out the other end of the room.

"We were both hiding from the people in the houses, the enemy villagers, Frodo called them. We had our hoods up so the Ring Wraiths couldn't see us. Then suddenly Frodo was being attacked by a Ring Wraith. He stood up, yelling and pretending to fight something. He was behind me—I wasn't looking at him. I think he might have stumbled backwards and tripped over the edge of the pavement. Then I heard a thump. I looked around, and a car was going by. I don't know how it got there. I saw Caleb, he was almost flying through the air after bouncing off the car."

"Then he was lying on the road. There was broken glass near him. His glasses got knocked off and broken, but I found them. I looked around for more cars. There was just one, and it had stopped. I called his name over and over. I wanted him to get off the road right away, to roll or crawl or something, but he just lay there. He didn't move, he didn't talk to me, and his eyes kept fluttering. At first, I thought he was faking, but then I got really scared." Eliza was breathing rapidly, and her words were coming in bursts.

"I didn't know what to do… If he wasn't going to move, I had to move him. I had to get him to the grass, where it was safer, so I dragged him. I tried grabbing under his armpits. I had to go backwards, pulling him. He was so heavy. I tried pulling on the shoulders of his coat, then I tried his armpits again. It was really hard… Nobody came to help… It seemed like nobody was near… I didn't know where Mom was. He wasn't waking up, just moving his eyelids a tiny bit."

Gasping now, Eliza was overtaken by sobs. Brooke put a hand on her arm. Eliza collected herself, took a deep breath and plunged on.

"Then, finally, some people came…they were too late to help me. They were asking me to go and get help… I went to get Aunt Dawn. Then she came back with me, and Mom was there, and there were sirens, and an ambulance and police cars and flashing lights… it was awful."

She turned to Brooke, her eyes brimming with tears. Brooke wiped Eliza's eyes and then clasped both her hands.

"You did the right thing. You were very brave, 'Liza. You were a loyal companion, just like Sam. I'm very proud of you. Your mom and dad are too." Brooke wrapped an arm around Eliza's shoulders and gave her a gentle squeeze.

Brooke surveyed the room, looking for a way to distract Eliza from the troubling scenes she had described. Brooke's gaze landed on a crafts table piled with supplies to entertain Dawn's young guests at Christmas. There was a jar of markers, another jar of pipe-cleaners, a bottle of craft glue and pads of paper in varying sizes.

"Caleb is in his own room now. The walls are pretty bare. Wouldn't it be cool to make some cards and drawings for him to see when he can open his eyes?"

Eliza followed her gaze to the craft table, and almost leapt into action, making a plan as she crossed the room. She first thought of a "get well" card, but then she found a pad of white drawing paper, and turned her mind to how to make a picture of the logo of Caleb's favourite hockey team, the Calgary Flames. Brooke helped by pulling up a Flames logo on her phone, and they got to work. While she coloured their picture, Eliza chattered happily about how surprised Caleb would be if this was the first thing he saw.

When the picture was finished, Brooke went upstairs to discover that the plan had changed: Dawn was settling the children into beds at her house, and had taken Doreen home. She had returned bringing Eliza's bag back so that Eliza, too, could sleep at Dawn and Tom's house.

On her way home, Brooke felt wrung out. From seeing Caleb in the Emergency Room to saying goodnight to Eliza, she felt completely exhausted, more than she usually felt from her busy shifts at the hospital. Her heart ached—for Eliza, especially.

On the following day Brooke was not scheduled to work, but she phoned her unit to find out which Child Life Worker would be on duty. She was put through to a worker named Erinn.

"Hi Erinn, it's Brooke Newsome calling, about one of your patients. He's an eleven-year-old from Saskatchewan, Caleb Pate."

"Hey Brooke, I heard he's your cousin. So sorry for your family!"

"Thanks, but not really *my* cousin. He's my boyfriend's cousin. But thanks. I've known the boy for a while. Everybody in Andrew's family has been in knots since it happened."

"Of course. It's so tough, the waiting."

"There's another thing: He has a nine-year-old sister who was there when it happened. She was alone with him for several minutes until help came. She's a bit distressed…"

"Understandably!" Erinn paused. "Are you asking me for something, Brooke?"

"Just a heads-up, really. You are probably going to see her today. Her mom might bring her in."

"Okay, I'll keep an eye out. Don't worry at all."

"It's just, well, these kids are from a tiny town in Saskatchewan. They don't have a lot of experience with city traffic, even paved roads. It seems like even the sirens and flashing lights are a very big deal for Eliza—that's her name, Eliza, or sometimes just Liza. Plus, you know there's that feeling that there was something else that she could have done or should have done… She seemed really wrecked last night. Just watch out for her, okay?"

Brooke felt a need to end her chat with Erinn as her emotions were threatening to take over.

"Got it. Don't worry, Brooke. I'm making a chart note, in case I'm not the one on duty when—what's the name? Eliza?—oh yes, here she is, mentioned in the chart: She pulled her big brother off the road? Wow!

Again, don't worry. What you are describing is common, in adults as well as children. We tend to go over and over the events, evaluating our own part, trying to make it come out differently. It's always on my radar. I'll definitely watch for Eliza and spend time with her."

Brooke signed off, feeling a bit of relief. Both Caleb and Eliza would get good care.

Erinn was indeed ready when Bettina and Eliza arrived later. Bruce returned to stay in Caleb's room at around eight in the morning so that Bettina could drive back to Brantford, get a shower and spend part of the day with the other children. In the afternoon she returned with Eliza and sent Bruce back to Brantford for a few hours.

Erinn took both Eliza and Bettina for a long chat, allowing Eliza to do some drawing if she chose to. They sat in the Child Life counselling office, where Erinn had some art supplies just for such occasions. Flipping through Caleb's chart, Erinn had absorbed the information about the family's Christian faith. As they all stood to bring the meeting to a close, Erinn allowed Eliza to leave the office first and make her way back to Caleb's room. She caught Bettina's eye, to hold her back for a private chat.

"I think you have already thought of this, but your prayers for healing should include Eliza as well as Caleb. What she has seen and done, well, she's a brave girl, but it's a lot for a child. She will need some time to process it."

"I did think about that," Bettina agreed. "She seems so strong, but that's just her way. Plus she looks grown up, for her age. Her father and I will certainly be praying for both of them, and watching Eliza carefully. Thank you."

"She's a sweet and lovely girl, and such a loyal friend for Caleb! I predict they will help each other get through this."

Bettina could only nod gratefully. She left the office and returned to Caleb's room, feeling God's hand of comfort on her shoulder.

CHAPTER EIGHT

FRIDAY DECEMBER 23—WAITING

D r. Ajani, a pediatric neurosurgeon, became a familiar face over the next four weeks for Bruce and Bettina. He was a striking figure, a tall Black man who filled the doorframe when he casually leaned in to check on his young patients. Soon after he had read Caleb's admission notes and test results, he had offered Caleb's parents his forecast that Caleb would make a full recovery, despite his unresponsive state and the signs of bleeding in his brain.

Although Bruce and Bettina found reassurance in these remarks, big questions about Caleb's future still hovered, like storm clouds. There were so many unknown factors when an injury occurred inside the skull. They couldn't help wondering when they would begin to see any sort of recovery at all, never mind a full recovery.

There was sunshine behind those clouds, for sure: Caleb was in the best children's hospital available, possibly the best in Canada. They had experienced amazing care and compassion already. Dozens of family members and friends, both nearby and far away, were providing support and prayers. Bruce and Bettina were humbled and grateful for the outpouring of love. It braced them for the long wait ahead.

Dr. Nikil Pai, a pediatrician, wrote the Daily Progress Note for Caleb on December 23. He mentions GCS, the Glasgow Coma Scale, giving Caleb a score of six, the same score assessed by the ambulance attendants, an alarmingly low rating. His note also included the omi-nous phrase "acute axonal injury." Although Bruce and Bettina had an early sense that things would be okay, these earliest medical tests sug-gested that things could easily have tipped the other way.

Dr. Ajani came by daily. On an early visit, he offered an illustration of the functions of the brain, which shed some light on the medical lingo in Caleb's charts. Dr. Ajani compared the three parts of brain function to a generator, wiring, and a set of lights. The generator was working, he said. Some of the lights worked. The wiring, however, was damaged, and would need time to heal. Dr. Ajani seemed fairly sure that the rest of the lights would work, eventually. He and his team began the work of controlling expectations: they needed Bruce and Bettina to understand that healing sometimes takes a lot of time, and a lot of work by the patient himself. There wasn't going to be a magic moment when Caleb suddenly woke up, spoke, got dressed and went home.

Axons are long, connecting nerve fibers inside the brain that can get stretched and damaged when the brain shifts or rotates inside its protective shell of the skull. Coma is a common result, and sometimes serious injury to brain function.

The rooms for patients in McMaster's PICU have a bed for parents or other visitors to spend the night, when necessary. The bed folds up into a chair during the day. In Caleb's room, the bed was, at first, occu-pied by either Bettina or Bruce. Later, other adults came in from time to time, to visit, or to hold the fort while Bruce and Bettina had a break. For every minute of the first forty-eight hours, the adults hoped and expected that Caleb might open his eyes, or speak to them. He did not.

Sometimes during the night he would move his arms and legs spontaneously, but his eyes remained closed. The fluttering-eyelids that Eliza had observed at the roadside was not present.

On December 23, Bettina sent the first of many text messages on Caleb's condition to the many relatives and friends, both in Ontario and Saskatchewan, who were eager to know how Caleb was doing.

So far, they stopped the sedation at 10. He has not opened his eyes yet but is moving everything well. Not following commands just yet. The neurosurgeon said he is improving but it could be up to 1-2 weeks before he really wakes up. Might need some therapy but they do expect a full recovery

They plan to take the breathing tube out soon.

The breathing tube frustrated Bettina. As a nurse, she understood its function, but as it had been many hours since the accident, she felt it should be removed. All signs indicated no damage to the cervical spine, therefore no paralysis. What if he began to wake up, and couldn't speak because of the tube in his throat? He wouldn't understand what was going on.

The staff may have been sympathetic, but they needed Caleb to respond to pain-sensitivity tests in his limbs, before removing the tube. This testing was the required diagnostic tool to rule out spinal cord damage. However, a comatose patient cannot reliably respond or react to the stimulation of his hands and feet. In addition, the respiratory technologists were extremely busy with child-patients whose needs were more urgent than Caleb's. The tube stayed.

Reducing the sedation enabled the medical people to observe Caleb's ability to move his limbs spontaneously, but, at first, their repeated requests, "Move your arm" or "Move your leg," got no reaction. He was not hearing, or could not comply. They would continue to wait.

In a lined notebook, Bettina began a log of each step in his treatment. At first there was no change in his condition. Then, slowly, incrementally, she noted tiny improvements.

Finally, in the late afternoon of December 23, his breathing tube was removed. He looked much more "normal," lying in bed without it, and could roll around more freely.

Bettina began to stack the business cards of his caregivers on the rolling tray-table in Caleb's room She also kept a journal of professional and family visitors. Owing to changing shifts, and holiday schedules, the faces of Caleb's care team kept shifting. She and Bruce would have rapidly lost track of who said what to them, but for their careful note-taking.

The care-giver list included two respiratory technologists, many registered nurses, a child life specialist, two or three different physiotherapists, occupational therapists, a social worker, and even a psychotherapist, not to mention pediatric neurosurgeons, fellows, residents and medical students.

Bettina was conversant with hospital shorthand and acronyms. Her notes, both in her journal and in bulletins to family, were sprinkled with the health-care version of alphabet soup: RT, RN, CL, PT, OT, and 'Psych.' She also logged the tests and scans to which Caleb was subjected, including X-ray (XR), computer-assisted tomography (CT) and magnetic resonance imaging (MRI), together with the medical terms that summarized findings. She wrote carefully and neatly. At her nursing job in Saskatchewan, chart notes were for medical teammates. At McMaster, they were addressed to Caleb, to be read with him when he was ready to ask questions about what had happened to him. When he was conscious and curious.

When not "if."

Bettina and Bruce took turns caring for the children during the day, each spending part of the day with Caleb, and some hours with the other children in Brantford. Bettina spent most nights at the hospital. Over the following week, both spent enough time at the hospital for the functions of all of Caleb's specialized workers to begin to fit into a recognizable pattern. It had only been a few days since the accident, but time was no longer marked in days; instead it passed in hours as they monitored the condition of their son and watched and waited for the improvements which would mean returning to a "normal life."

CHAPTER NINE

SATURDAY, DECEMBER 24—TRANSFER

On December 24, Caleb began to show signs of improvement. He was far from fully conscious, but he was also deemed to be out of danger. His recovery had become a waiting game: waiting for brain-swelling to subside, waiting for the stretched or bruised axons (nerves) to repair themselves as best they could, waiting for him to open his eyes and offer just the suggestion of a smile or a grin.

After sixteen hours, the saline solution administered to help reduce brain swelling was discontinued. The sedation continued while the breathing tube was in place, but after twenty-four hours, the tube was removed and sedation ceased. When these medications ended, he received some Tylenol for a few days, as he was moaning from time to time. It was difficult to know whether the moaning was due to pain.

Apart from these modest steps, no drugs or significant interventions were required. Only time. He was transferred out of Intensive Care, to a regular in-patient ward. Bettina sent out another bulletin:

> *Caleb is on a regular Pediatric floor now. He continues to move his arms and legs. Today he moved his eyes when they did a pupil check! Every day we see something new*

and improving! We continue to pray for Caleb to wake up and for the swelling in his brain to decrease.

We are so grateful to everyone for your prayers, support, and the love you are showing to all of us! 🙏

As the first days dragged on, more members of the extended family became acquainted with caregiver chair-bed in Caleb's room. Often, aunts or uncles or cousins sat or napped in the chair, while Caleb, mostly motionless and silent, slept in the dimly lit room. For several days, there was still no sign that he was awake.

For Christmas Eve, Dawn Pate took over at around 8:30 pm and stayed so that Bettina and Bruce could get back to Grandma's house and put the children to bed. Bettina's bulletin for the day:

Dawn is staying with Caleb tonight so we could take Grandma to church and have Christmas in the morning. She is too kind!

I think we will take all the kids and maybe Grandma to see Caleb in the morning

Caleb's room, with a window looking across a courtyard, had started to look like a campsite or a garage sale. This was unavoidable: it was a second, or perhaps third, home for Bruce and Bettina as well as a place to receive their many visitors. There was a tiny mini-fridge in one corner, and along the wide windowsill there were apples and donuts, many gifts of food, piles of coats and hats, books, knapsacks, cards and balloons.

Bruce and Bettina kept a Bible open on the small counter beside the sink. Other books, notebooks, pens, snacks, drinks and food trays filled most of the portable table, which Caleb was not yet able to use for meals. Cards and drawings made by Eliza, Ethan, and Lukas were taped to the wall and doors, along with medical memos about what to expect from brain-injury patients. The logo of the Calgary Flames (Caleb's favourite hockey team) was displayed prominently so that Caleb would see it as soon as his eyes opened.

Although the room seemed like it couldn't hold anything else, Christmas was about to arrive. And with it, more of everything.

THE TWELVE DAYS
OF CHRISTMAS

CHAPTER TEN

SUNDAY DECEMBER 25 —CHRISTMAS DAY

Life went on around Caleb, as he seemed to sleep endlessly, but it was not always a deep sleep. Bettina and Bruce could recognize small but significant changes. Bettina sent out another bulletin to friends and relatives, listing some of these clues:

> *Today Caleb is making more facial expressions and his heart rate went up a bit more when we all arrived this morning. He knows we are here! He is also making some noises in his throat, kind of like moans, which are new since yesterday.*
>
> *The hospital has a large gift bag for Christmas for him to open as well as a large bag for all the siblings! We continue to receive excellent care here!*

His brothers and sister came to visit, hugging him while he lay in the bed. It was the first time they had seen their brother dressed in a hospital gown but otherwise looking the same as if he were at home, sleeping late.

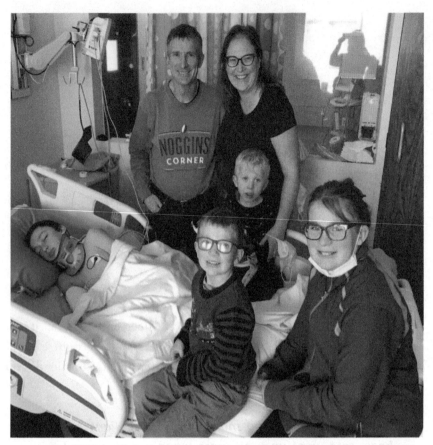

3 Bruce, Bettina with Lukas, Ethan, and Eliza in Caleb's room.

Eliza and her little brothers expected a response. It was heartbreaking for Bettina and Bruce as the children called his name, whispered in his ear and generally tried their best to wake him. They brought his Christmas presents, still wrapped, and were very disappointed that he could not unwrap them, or even look at them.

All of Caleb's presents, those from family as well as a huge bag of presents from his care team, were soon crammed into his room. There were wrapped gifts under the counter-top and sink, on the windowsill and in every available nook in his room, awaiting that day for which his parents prayed, when he would be able to open them himself. He slept on.

Later that day, his caregivers encouraged Caleb to respond, trying various commands and tests. "Caleb, can you move this arm? Now this one?" At times like this, his eyes seemed to be open, just a sliver, not entirely open. To encourage him, in case bright lights hurt, the room lights were rarely turned on. The large window was the main light source.

The physiotherapist pointed out that Caleb was processing what he was hearing and seemed ready to try hard to respond to commands. Bettina was pleased about this breakthrough moment, but now a new issue presented itself: his eleven-year-old body could not get sufficient nourishment through intra-venous drips.

Nutrition was essential for the healing and restoration of damaged tissues. Until he could demonstrate an ability to suck on a straw, swallow, and eventually to chew, Caleb would need a feeding tube. It would be inserted through the nose and gently guided down Caleb's throat, avoiding the windpipe. The upper end of the tube was attached to a bag hanging from a pole near the bed. The bag held a liquid that looked like café au lait, but probably wasn't. Neither Caleb nor anyone else tasted this liquid as it dripped slowly into his stomach. Quite soon, this tube would become one more thing that Caleb would resist. For now, though, it could not be avoided.

> *We continue to pray for God's perfect timing for Caleb to wake up. If his brain needs more time to heal, then we want to be patient. Although I did have a dream last night that he opened his eyes!*
>
> *Thank you for your continued prayers, love and support! We are truly humbled at the outpouring of love from all of you!*

CHAPTER ELEVEN

MONDAY DECEMBER 26 — MIDDLE EARTH

Monday was a day of more incremental progress. Mindy, a physiotherapist, and Heather, a registered nurse, encouraged Caleb to sit up on the edge of his bed. He managed this, with assistance, although his eyes were not fully open. Uncle Tom stayed in Caleb's room for much of the day and watched these gradual steps.

Bettina composed another text-message news bulletin, in what would become a long series:

> *A physiotherapist was in yesterday afternoon and today and said that Caleb is really trying hard to follow commands and move the parts she asks him to. She even got him to raise his arm and then give a "hug" to me yesterday. ⏃ I got three hugs!*
>
> *We continue to wait and pray for his eyes to open on his own. When they check his pupils, he is moving his eyes back and forth more and that is a good sign. Once he is awake, we will have a better idea of whether rehab will be weeks or months. Each kid is so different!*

Bruce's brother Tom and sister-in-law Dawn are taking turns with Caleb today since our other kids need us! We have spent the morning building Lego and playing with Christmas gifts. It has been good to spend time at Grand-ma's but I am torn and want to be with Caleb too.

Thank you for your continued prayers and support for all of us! We are most grateful!

Bettina brought Ethan for a visit in the evening. She was delighted to discover that Caleb's cervical collar (neck brace) had been removed, another milestone that made him look more normal to his family and his visitors. It also made him more comfortable when lying in bed.

By this time, all family members and visitors were cured of the notion, encouraged by television dramas, that comatose patients regain consciousness suddenly and pick up conversations where they left off. That wasn't what was happening with Caleb, or at least not yet. He was no longer in a deep coma, but he was also not fully conscious, not present. He was somewhere in between, a place between the coma and the world where his parents and family lived. It was as if he had stayed in the mythical land of his favourite book, Tolkien's *Lord of the Rings*, an imaginary place where he and Eliza often played: Middle Earth.

CHAPTER TWELVE

TUESDAY, DECEMBER 27

Aunt Dawn spent the night in Caleb's room. On Tuesday, Bettina and Eliza shared an experience that was new for both of them: they went to the Brantford Police Headquarters, where each gave a statement. Eliza met with a female officer specializing in dealing with children. Bettina met with one of the officers who had attended at the accident scene.

Days later the police advised Bruce and Bettina that the driver would not be charged. Finding no evidence of alcohol, excessive speed or distracted driving, the investigators evaluated the possibility that the accident could have been avoided. Their conclusion was that, because the children were hiding in the shadows, what happened was not foreseeable and therefore probably not avoidable. The driver described a shadowy shape appearing so suddenly that he wasn't even sure it was a person until he walked back and saw a boy on the ground.

The officers had to base their opinions on tire marks, Caleb's bruises and the other circumstances. No one but the driver had witnessed the actual moment of impact. Even Eliza had her back turned.

The police determined that the driver had behaved reasonably before, during, and after the incident. He was watching the road and saw nothing until it was too late to avoid impact. He had less than a second to react. He braked and swerved just as Caleb's hip contacted the car. He was travelling within the normal range of speed for that road. The investigators found that none of the elements of careless or dangerous driving were present. There was no criminal charge or even traffic infraction that made sense to the officers. However, this left the door open for Bruce and Bettina to sue the driver in civil court.

Bruce and Bettina made a few phone calls and determined that Saskatchewan's provincial insurance scheme would cover all of their travel and parking expenses and Caleb's medical costs both in Ontario and when they returned home. They would have minimal costs for accommodation and meals because they had so many relatives nearby. Although they consulted a lawyer in Hamilton, they concluded that there was no need to engage the driver's Ontario insurance.

The families of young patients without a network of local relatives and friends can stay at a free residence, Ronald McDonald House, near McMaster Hospital. Thanks to the proximity of Bruce's family members, they did not even consider bunking in at McDonald House. Bruce and Bettina felt fortunate to be in a position to weather this storm without the added stress of financial or legal worries, or even feeling isolated and alone. On the contrary, they had wrap-around care.

Bettina's message for the fifth day of their ordeal conveys the difficulty of waiting, not knowing, and trusting that Caleb will wake up, when he is ready:

Today the physio even sat him on the edge of the bed while supporting him. Every now and then his eyes are slightly open so we see a little bit of eyeball ☺

Conversations with various members of his team today reminded us that the road to full recovery will likely be months of rehab. But again that will be easier to know once he wakes up. This reminds us of the need to be patient 🙏

Medically, Caleb has stabilized. His sodium levels were good so the intravenous line has been removed. They were able to increase his feeds by nasal tube which is good. He's responding a bit more each day which is also encouraging. They expect that it will be another 1-2 weeks before he's awake. The waiting is definitely not easy but we continue to pray for full and complete healing in his mind and body 🙏 thank you for joining us in prayer and for your support!

CHAPTER THIRTEEN

WEDNESDAY, DECEMBER 28

Bettina spent the night at the hospital and woke up there on December 28. Wednesday was about to deliver a big boost to the family's understanding of brain trauma and to Caleb's progress.

Bettina describes it, opening with a Bible verse:

> *Today I wanted to share something I read to Caleb this morning and then give you the amazing update from his therapy session this morning!*
>
> *"I believe that I shall see the goodness of the Lord in the land of the living. Wait for the Lord; be strong, and let your heart take courage; wait for the Lord!" Psalm 27:13-14*
>
> *It wasn't too long after reading that when the physio and occupational therapists came in. They put some pants on Caleb and we got his shoes on. He was able to sit at the edge of the bed. He stood up when they asked him to...he opened his eyes a bit and looked right at me. He gave me three strong hugs! Then the most amazing thing was that he walked down the hall!! He tried to hold his head up and he had his eyes half open some of the time! He walked about 15 meters, took a rest, and then walked another*

20-25 meters! I got to be right at his side while he walked.
It was truly amazing and we were all in tears! Tears of joy!
Now he is sitting up in a special reclining wheelchair with
sunglasses on 😎. We are completely amazed, thrilled, and
grateful! God gave us another miracle today!

Thank you for keeping us in your prayers and for not giving
up! 🙏 We continue to anticipate Caleb being fully awake!

Bettina, her eyes still streaming tears of joy, called Bruce to tell him the wonderful news. Although Caleb's level of consciousness was a bit ambiguous, with his eyes only partially open, and frequently closing, he was still showing signs of consciousness about a week ahead of what had been forecast by Dr. Ajani and his team.

Eliza also visited in the evening, getting a ride to Hamilton with her cousin Erica. Caleb seemed to recognize who was there and sat up on the bed on his own initiative. His eyes were half-open. His face registered no emotion. Despite this, the act of sitting up and the partly open eyes were signs of hope that Eliza had been craving. She had been impatient to see her brother returning to normal a lot sooner. She reluctantly accepted that this was the best he could do, for now.

From this milestone onward, Caleb was encouraged to spend time sitting up every few hours. The wheelchair was a deluxe model, sized for him, and capable of tilting like a reclining armchair. Caleb was not permitted to stand by himself while the chair was positioned for him. Once in it, he was buckled in securely. The care team took extreme caution to avoid the possibility that a brain-injured patient like Caleb might fall and hit his head while transferring to and from the chair, nor did he walk anywhere without a team-member at his elbow. However, he had shown that he could walk, and that he was happy about it. After a long wait for only meagre signs of progress, Caleb's assisted walking was a leap forward and offered his parents immeasurable joy. And it was only the beginning.

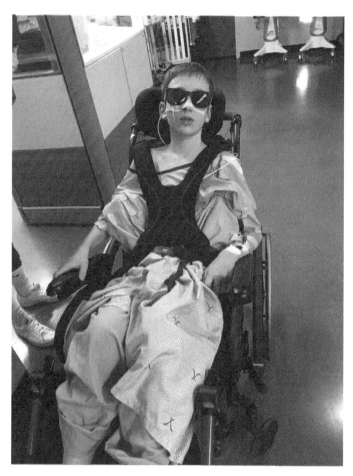

4 Caleb in the rehab wheelchair with protective sunglasses.

CHAPTER FOURTEEN

THURSDAY DECEMBER 29 — ONE WEEK AFTER ARRIVING AT MCMASTER

The next day Caleb was able to demonstrate unambiguously that he was aware of who was in the room. When Bettina arrived in the morning to take over from Bruce, Caleb sat up in his bed.

Shortly afterward, Asha, an occupational therapist, came to Caleb's bedside and encouraged him to sit, then to stand. She eased him into the wheelchair. Once he was settled, she tried to interest him in sipping some water or apple juice but he would not drink. Asha would keep trying this until she got the desired responses. If he were really waking up, he would be thirsty, he would be able to taste, and he would be eager to swallow. Caleb's brain circuits for these normal, daily functions seemed not to be repaired yet. Nonetheless, she could tell that he knew what she was asking him to do, and that was a positive sign, even if his answer was "no."

A bulletin posted in Caleb's room noted that brain-injured patients expend huge amounts of energy to do tasks that were previously effortless: sitting up, walking, doing exercises in response to his physiotherapist—all of these activities would exhaust him. He was napping frequently.

For seven days, Bettina had been reporting on Caleb's condition to an ever-widening community of support. In return, the first circle relatives, community friends, and work colleagues sent inquiries and messages of support, passing the news on to others. Soon Bettina and Bruce were very busy reading and responding to messages. Bettina printed out some of them to paste into the journal that she was creating for Caleb.

Bettina's bulletins often included a lot of medical detail for the benefit of the many Pate relatives who worked in health care, and for her teammates at Cypress Regional Hospital in Swift Current, Saskatchewan. Prior to the accident, Bettina worked just a few shifts each month at the hospital in Swift Current, and regarded those days as "rest and relaxation," compared to the pace of being a mother with four children at home.

Without knowing how long Caleb would need to be in hospital, she and Bruce had begun to look ahead to when one of them would have to take Eliza, Ethan, and Lukas back to Saskatchewan. Weeks earlier, they had booked their return tickets to Regina for January 3, which was the normal length of stay at Grandma's. A longer stay might cease to be fun for Grandma Doreen, as well as for Eliza, who would miss her school and friends. Depending on what was in Caleb's future, they might have to have one parent return home for a couple of weeks, then switch around with the other parent going home. They prepared mentally for the possibility that this would go on for months. They planned that Bettina would return with the children first.

"Home" was Gloryview, their farm in Saskatchewan.

Would they return to a normal home life anytime soon? So far, with abundant help from family, they had been able to give the other kids a relatively normal Christmas visit to Grandma's and to the homes of various aunts and uncles.

The children had new toys, and Brantford was enjoying the snowiest winter in years. Only Eliza would be disappointed if they had to stay a little longer than expected. But that was significant. Eliza was already caring the burden of having been with Caleb when the accident happened and struggled with seeing him appear to be so damaged. Bettina wanted to get Eliza back to Saskatchewan where Bettina's parents, Manfred and Renate Kurschner, were watching and waiting prayerfully from afar.

Bettina's older son, Micah, Bruce's stepson, was also anxious to be kept in the loop. Although he lived and worked in Swift Current, twenty-five minutes from Gloryview, he came home frequently to visit the family. Micah was missing all of them, and was worried about Caleb.

Repeatedly Bettina thanked their large group of supporters when she composed her daily bulletins. She felt buoyed up by the knowledge that so many people cared and were praying for Caleb and for the other members of the family. It was becoming impossible to send individual replies to all the texts and emails she was receiving, so she and Bruce had begun to send out one daily bulletin to everyone on their list. Bettina's original punctuation demonstrates how excited she was by each small measure of progress.

Update for Dec 29, 2022

In a few hours it will be a week since the accident. Crazy!!

We want to just share our appreciation for all your prayers and supports!! The entire medical, therapy, and nursing team here keeps telling us that Caleb is doing well!

....

With Physiotherapy (PT), he got back to the edge of the bed. He assisted in getting himself dressed in his own clothes and walked down a long hallway with an assistant accompanying him! Today Bruce got to see it too!!

I was able to help by getting him glasses. The gentleman at the store found a frame that fit his current lenses perfectly!! And the frame is red- his favourite color!! Another little miracle ☺.

As we continue to journey with Caleb, we are excited about the little things that he is doing each day. God is good and He is faithful and we are grateful to all of you as well as the excellent medical/nursing/therapy team here at McMaster Children's Hospital and to our local family members who are helping us in many ways! ❦

CHAPTER FIFTEEN

FRIDAY DECEMBER 30

Caleb's communications with others, although not yet verbal, continued to surge forward on Friday. He could not be considered to be fully awake yet: he had made no attempts at verbalizing and had not accepted any liquids other than tiny sips of water. Even so, the gains in his awareness and responses to others showed steady progress in restored brain function.

> *Update for Dec 30, 2022*
>
> *"May you be strong with all the strength that comes from His glorious power, and may you be prepared to endure everything with patience, while joyfully giving thanks to the Father..." Colossians 1:11-12a*
>
> *This is what I read with Caleb this morning. We've seen some more new things again so that is exciting!! Last night when Bruce came in, Caleb sat up in the bed and reached his arms out to give Bruce a hug.*
>
> *This morning, our nurse from Pediatric Intensive Care came to say hi. As he was leaving, I asked Caleb to wave good-bye and he did! Then he gave the nurse a high five too!*

Caleb has been walking well today. We have seen his eyes open more often and he is definitely doing more purposeful movement. He took a small sip of water with the Occupational Therapist today.

He just walked the long hall twice, almost on his own (using a walker) and minimal assist!! Walking is definitely his favourite thing to do so far ☺

We are encouraged and grateful! Thank you again for your continued prayers for full healing and recovery!! 🙏

Once Caleb began to recognize his visitors, and responded to them, his neurosurgeon's daily appearance became a useful counterpoint, to put Caleb's progress in perspective. Each day on his rounds, Dr. Ajani, would read Caleb's medical chart while outside the room, then step into the room and ask Caleb the same question: "Have you seen me before?" Dr. Anjani's booming voice and imposing presence were not easy to forget. Nonetheless, Caleb would shake his head "no," day after day. He knew family members, but he was not yet forming new memories of each day.

By this simple question, Dr. Ajani could gauge whether Caleb's brain circuits involved in recording and retrieving recent memories were functioning. So far, the answer was "no."

CHAPTER SIXTEEN

SATURDAY DECEMBER 31, 2022

Update for Dec 31, 2022

So crazy that we are on the last day of the year already!! Next year is full of promise and fresh starts and new beginnings!

Cousins came by the hospital today and shared this verse with Caleb:

"Do not fear, for I am with you, do not be afraid, for I am your God; I will strengthen you, I will help you, I will uphold you with My victorious right hand."

Isaiah 41:10

Eliza came with me to hang out with Caleb today! We got here at 10 and physio was ready to work with him!

Eliza and I both got hugs when he first stood up!

He walked the entire ward with his walker today with only a short rest. He was able to keep his balance fairly well, and the physio was just holding his back lightly. He did really well! But you can tell that all of this moving in the past few days has really worn him out.

He is keeping his eyes open more during his walks and looking ahead to avoid obstacles. He is also following commands more quickly and consistently!! It is hard to believe that less than a week ago, he was basically just sleeping in bed and moving his legs and arms around. He has really come so far!!

After sitting up in his wheelchair for a while, it was time to go back to bed. Eliza wanted to show Caleb something she had made for him and he looked right at her and then the small fish bowl we made with clay! Very intentional! Then he willingly lay down and pulled the blanket up over his shoulders. ☺ He also took his glasses off before going soundly to sleep.

We plan to get Caleb a shower this afternoon so I hope that will feel good for him.

These don't seem like big deals for most people but these are gigantic steps for Caleb this week!!

Thank you for your continued prayers for Caleb's mind to fully heal and return to being able to do all the things he did before ☺☐🙏

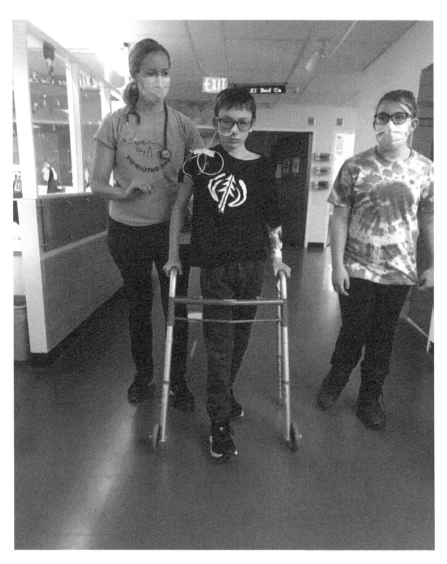

5 Caleb with his physiotherapist and Eliza strolling in the hospital corridor.

CHAPTER SEVENTEEN

SUNDAY JANUARY 1, 2023

Update for Jan 1, 2023

"I can do all things through Christ who gives me strength."

Philippians 4:13

What a great promise for a new year!!

Today we all came to see Caleb after church. Bruce had stayed the night at the hospital, and I took Grandma and the kids to our cousin's church. They prayed for Caleb and the kids each got to light one of the advent candles in honor of Caleb. It was a moving moment!

Today Caleb got on a trike that he pedalled around the hospital "block" (330m)!! He did the pedalling and steering and had his eyes partly open! It was fun to see him getting further on his own steam ☺ and I think he enjoyed it too!

Some of you have been asking about travel and therapy plans so I will include that today:

Bruce will stay with Caleb until we see what would be the best long-term therapy for him. Options include Toronto, Saskatoon, Edmonton, Calgary. We want to access the program that would be the best for Caleb in the long run. Because of the holidays, it's hard to get in touch with people so we will probably know better at the end of next week.

I plan to bring Eliza, Ethan, and Lukas home again on Tuesday. The kids need to get back into their routines and school. It will be hard to leave Caleb behind but perhaps Bruce and I will take turns being with Caleb once we know the plan better.

We remain humbled and grateful at the support, love, and prayers you are all giving on behalf of Caleb!! We look forward to many amazing things this new year! Happy New Year from all of us!!

That night, while a cousin was staying with Caleb to give Bruce a night off, Caleb pulled out his nasal feeding tube. Twice. Re-inserting it was a tricky process, requiring an X-ray to confirm that the tube has entered the stomach, as opposed to the windpipe. Before it could be hooked up to allow the liquid nutrients to flow, a portable X-ray machine would confirm that the tube was not going into the wrong place. Each time Caleb pulled it out, it took two staff members several minutes to re-insert it, which was challenging, particularly during the night shift when less staff were available.

The first time Caleb pulled out the tube, it could be seen as an accident. After the staff laboured to re-install it, and he pulled it out a second time, Caleb was signaling that he found the nasal tube an irritant, and had sufficient coordination to tug on it until it came out. Pulling out the tube must have caused Caleb some discomfort, and having it re-inserted would not have been pleasant either. It was a tough night for Caleb and for his companion.

Over the next two days, Caleb's resistance to tube-feeding was a game-changer. His healing process would be diminished without adequate nutrition, and he could not yet eat. Team members wondered if the course of his recovery had started to go sideways.

CHAPTER EIGHTEEN

MONDAY JANUARY 2

The pediatric unit had a wide variety of resources and activities for children like Caleb. The tricycle that Caleb first rode "around the block" of hospital corridors on New Year's Day was no ordinary tricycle—it had to be quite large to work for a gangly eleven-year-old. It was low to the ground, with big wheels and a recumbent-style of saddle. This design made tipping over virtually impossible, thus, balance was not an issue and cornering was not risky. Caleb seemed to enjoy himself while demonstrating pedaling and steering, and awareness of the space he was in. In vain, Bettina watched for his usual broad smile or a proud and cocky grin, but no emotions flickered over his features.

The tricycle was just the beginning: in the therapy room, the physiotherapists had several activities that made therapy into fun and games. The hospital even had a scaled-down hockey net and practice pucks for floor hockey.

Update for Jan 2, 2023

"I pray that, according to the riches of His glory, He may grant that you may be strengthened in your inner being with power through His Spirit..." Ephesians 3:16

Wow! What a day! I have to admit I was a bit discouraged this morning when we heard that Caleb had pulled his feeding tube twice in the night. They did get it reinserted finally and he got his feeds but he was quite sleepy until about 11:30. I did also tell him that I was leaving tomorrow and that was hard to do.

The neurosurgeon encouraged me again by saying he will be ok ☺ He also said that the Bloorview Kids' Rehabilitation Hospital[1] in Toronto is the best facility for Caleb (the best in Canada) and so he would work at getting Caleb admitted there ASAP! He ordered an MRI of his brain which was completed today.

Then OT came to try some food and Caleb even fed himself a few bites of yogurt! She stocked our little fridge in the room with snacks for him!

Then PT came...Caleb went for a short walk to the nurses' desk and waved at the nurses using his left hand! That is amazing because he hasn't been using that hand as much. We went to the therapy room where Caleb held a hockey stick and shot some pucks in the net! They went in every time! Then he also rode the bike another lap around the hospital. Amazing!!

He is now resting and having a well-deserved nap.

I am fully amazed to see how Caleb does something new each day!

His nurse today is the same nurse we had when he first came to this floor. She has said so many times today how Caleb's progress is awesome!! We are so encouraged by the amazing staff here who are rooting for him and also for the amazing team of family and friends praying for him everywhere!! Thank you!!

---

[1] Holland Bloorview Children's Rehabilitation Hospital, commonly known as "Bloorview".

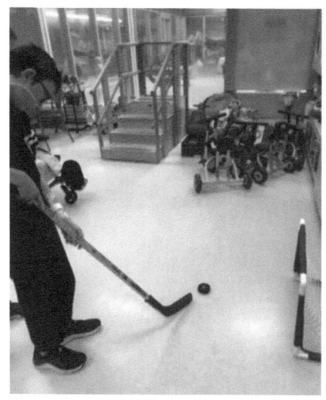

Miniature hockey in the physio room.

Also on that day, Caleb began indicating his wishes and needs by pointing. He could indicate the door to the bathroom, to request help in getting there. When he was tired of sitting in his wheelchair, he would point to the bed. At this stage he could stand by himself, but was strapped into the chair to prevent him from trying to stand without stabilization from a nurse or therapist.

The occupational therapist created situations for Caleb to make a decision and communicate with her: she held up a small pudding and half-cup yogurt container where Caleb could see them, and waited for him to indicate a preference, by a nod or a wave, almost in toddler-fashion. This interaction would have taken a healthy Caleb no time at all, or he would have immediately responded, "Both." But for Middle-Earth Caleb, this level of decision-making and gesturing was hard work.

When Bruce came to the hospital at around 8:30 pm to take the overnight shift, Caleb pointed at the television, to let his dad know that he wanted to watch. All week, the International Ice Hockey Federation Junior Men's Tournament had been televised from Montreal and Moncton. Various relatives, when they visited, had kept track of the tournament on phones or tablets while staying in Caleb's room, and talked about the tournament among themselves. Caleb was now awake enough to be interested.

Hockey was back on his radar!

CHAPTER NINETEEN

~~~~~~

MONDAY JANUARY 2—POSTSCRIPT

Tuesday was Bettina's travel day. Before Bruce drove the others to the airport in Toronto, they gathered the children in Caleb's room for goodbye hugs. Photos of that day show Caleb strapped into his wheelchair holding his youngest brother. His eyelids are not fully open, his face shows no expression, yet he appears to have one arm around little Lukas, who is sitting in his lap. Ethan and Eliza cling to either side of his wheelchair. It was the children's last time to see him, other than by Facetime, for about six weeks.

Bettina added this PostScript to her message for the day:

> *Thank you for your patience. I know many of you have been praying for us as we travelled home today and I wasn't able to answer all your messages. We got home safely at 8:30 tonight and the kids are all happy to be home. ☺ thank you for your messages and prayers!*
>
> *My highlight today is that Caleb gave us a little smile and there was some light in his eyes!! We each got beautiful hugs from him as well!*

Bettina was overcome with emotion during the last farewell hugs that she and the children gave Caleb. She commented on being greeted that day with a slight smile, so Caleb's failure or inability to show sadness at her departure must have stung just a little. In a later interview with Caleb, he revealed that he was not sufficiently awake on January 2 to grasp matters like distance, separation or even why both parents were seldom in the room at the same time.

Bettina and the children arrived home in Saskatchewan to an outpouring of love and concern from her rural community, expressed in gifts of food left in her kitchen. Her parents had been on hand to receive the gifts, sent in anticipation of her return. She trudged into her kitchen, laden with luggage, and found baked goods and casseroles jamming her freezer and kitchen counters. Amazed at the generosity of friends, neighbours and church members, she realized she might not need to worry about groceries or cooking for several days. It was like being hugged by fifty or a hundred people all at once: slightly smothering, but just what she needed!

CHAPTER TWENTY

TUESDAY JANUARY 3

Bruce took over the writing and sending of some of the news updates, once Bettina was home in Stewart Valley. Like Bettina, he often included a Bible text, to serve as a theme for the day. Here's Bruce:

> *"The Lord watch between you and me, when we are absent one from the other." Genesis 31:49*
>
> *Bettina, Eliza, Ethan, and Lukas got to the hospital this morning to spend some time with Caleb. Cousin Ann came at 10 am to watch Caleb, while I took the gang to the Toronto airport where we said our goodbye's.*
>
> *Everyone at the hospital is very impressed and surprised at how fast Caleb is progressing. Dr Ajani says he is ready to go for rehab to Bloorview where they would work on his speech and coordination. Very optimistic doctor. My kinda guy.*
>
> *We are looking forward to God's continuing healing of Caleb.*

There was a possibility that Caleb would repeatedly pull out his nasal tube overnight, as he had during the night of January 1. With this concern in mind, his caregivers increased their efforts to get him to take food by mouth. Caleb had demonstrated that he could swallow yogurt, and even could grasp a spoon. These activities must have been tiring for him. Even with someone else feeding him, he only consumed half of a tiny yogurt cup at a time, before resting.

An occupational therapist and a nurse brought a variety of foods to tempt him. At first, he ate small quantities of yogurt or applesauce. When he lost interest in these, it was hard to tell if he was exhausted, or found the taste and sensation unappealing. Then the therapist showed him a frozen fruit-juice bar. After only a moment, he pointed at the frozen treat.

Up to this point Caleb's face had not been expressive, other than the brief smile Bettina had mentioned. Those circuits showed few signs of being reconnected. But when he opened his mouth to receive the frozen juice treat, his eyes widened, and he sucked on it involuntarily. It seemed as if he had forgotten that anything could be that cold. A decision was required immediately: was this a good or bad thing? In a matter of seconds, he had clearly made his decision ("good thing!") but became exhausted before he succeeded in sucking on it for more than a few swallows. The therapist took it from him and made a mental note: introduce ice cream next.

Dr. Ajani put the challenge in simple terms: if Caleb could be encouraged to consume one litre of any fluids, including pudding, yogurts, Jello, frozen treats, milk juice or water, the feeding tube would be discontinued. If, on the other hand, he was not getting enough fluids, the hose for the nose would return. For the first stage of this challenge, Dr. Ajani was not at all concerned about Caleb's caloric intake or, indeed, whether he consumed any nutrients. The goal was basic: fluids, 1000 millilitres of anything. It is unlikely that Caleb heard or understood this challenge, but for Bruce, the occupational therapists and the nurses, it was "game on."

On the first day of this campaign, January 3, Caleb accomplished only about a quarter of Dr. Ajani's target, managing to swallow small amounts of yogurt or pudding at each meal. In the evening, his nurses brought another nasal tube, with the intention of constantly dripping nutrients into his stomach overnight. They tried five times to insert it. He resisted. Sedation did not help.

If Caleb thought he had won that round, he was actually hurting the cause and worrying his team.

At this point, Caleb weighed about 36.5 kilograms, about 80 pounds. He had lost three pounds since admission, not surprising considering how long he had been unconscious. Nonetheless, weight loss was inconsistent with a good recovery. Healing requires rest but also takes energy from the body. Something had to change.

That same evening the medical team decided that, as a temporary alternative, intravenous fluids could be administered overnight. They would find a solution to the problem in the morning.

For better or worse, Caleb had made his wishes abundantly clear. No nose tube. He seemed happy and slept soundly that night. Could he have been savouring his small victory, or was he still not in control of his actions?

CHAPTER TWENTY-ONE

WEDNESDAY JANUARY 4

Over the next few days, with Bettina in Saskatchewan, Bruce fell into a routine of living at the hospital except for a few hours in the late afternoon, when another family member would show up stay in Caleb's room so that Bruce could go to Brantford and eat dinner with his mother. Bruce would return around eight o'clock, and compose his own bulletins, to supplement Bettina's.

Caleb, meanwhile, had discovered, or re-discovered, FaceTime, a program that allowed him to see Bettina's face, while they used Bruce's cellphone in Hamilton and Bettina's cellphone in Stewart Valley to make the call. At first, he did not speak, but Bettina was able to encourage him, ask him questions, read and pray over the phone.

This daily phone contact with Caleb enabled Bettina to continue to write up news bulletins. For January 4, Bettina wrote this:

> *"The Lord bless you and keep you; the Lord make his face shine upon you and be gracious unto you; the Lord lift up his countenance upon you and give you his peace."*
>
> *Numbers 6:24-26*

This is the way I tuck each kid into bed and what I would say whenever I left Caleb for the evening. Yes, it is hard to be away, but we were able to have a good FaceTime session this morning. He was really concentrating and engaged as I read one of our devotions to him. At one point there was a question. He shook his head "no" because he didn't know the answer.

Caleb's challenge these days is to avoid the feeding tube being put back in! He fought hard to avoid it. But now he needs to make up the calories and protein he needs to sustain and to heal. The dietician and OT are working hard to make special milk shakes for him to drink so he can have the calories he needs.

The other prayer request would be his speech. We know it will come in time, and he is getting good at communicating with gestures. He knows how to ask for his glasses and has enjoyed watching a little of the World Junior Hockey Championships ☺.

Thank you for your continued prayers and partnership with us! We can feel God's peace on us because of your prayers and because of the hope we have in Him!

This was also the day that Caleb's team introduced ice cream to his diet, providing Bruce with a breakthrough moment. His decision to mix peanut butter cups and bits of brownie from the hospital tray into the melting ice cream wasn't just a random idea. It was the recipe for Moose Tracks ice cream, Caleb's hands-down favourite flavour.

Bruce was going to exploit Caleb's ice cream passion in ways that many eleven-year-olds can only dream about: Caleb would have ice-cream morning, noon and night, if that's what it took. And not just any flavour. Moose Tracks.

CHAPTER TWENTY-TWO

THURSDAY JANUARY 5
TO FRIDAY, JANUARY 6

A message composed by Bettina, with Bruce's notes, describes the new routine:

January 5 and 6 update

Mark 11:22-24

Then Jesus said to the disciples, "Have faith in God. I tell you the truth, you can say to this mountain, 'May you be lifted up, thrown into the sea,' and it will happen. But you must really believe it will happen and have no doubt in your heart. I tell you, you can pray for anything and if you believe that you've received it, it will be yours."

God has answered our prayers and continues to answer them.

Caleb enjoyed having his Moose Tracks ice cream for breakfast, lunch and supper. He even fed himself and lifted up the bowl to his mouth so he could get every drop. He met his daily calorie intake for the day and he did not need to be hooked up to an intravenous line overnight.

Sarah, one of his PTs, last saw him on Tuesday and was amazed at the improvements he has made in the last two days. She says the knitting of the brain's fibres is happening very fast. The messages are going through. His walking has greatly improved and she did not find any deficits. She is seeing progress in all his motor functions. She could not believe that he sleeps through the night. She says it is very uncommon. Usually brain injury patients are very restless and agitated.

While the neurosurgeon was in, Caleb gave him a little wave and then got up out of bed to go pee. Dr. Ajani was impressed. He asked Caleb if he has seen him before and Caleb shook his head, "No." He said he will come back tomorrow and ask him the same question.

Thanks again for lifting up Caleb in prayer. We are thankful for you and for God. God is good!

Bruce put out a request for the next visitors to bring in pails of ice cream. There was a Ronald McDonald Foundation suite just around the corner from Caleb's room, where parents enjoy a coffee break and decompress. This room had a full-sized fridge with a freezer where Bruce could store Caleb's lifeline, Moose Tracks.

Of course the medical team made sure that there were other items available, such as bananas, milk-shakes and yogurt. Ice cream was to be used as the incentive to get Caleb to eat other things. This pattern continued as Bruce and the therapists introduced other foods, and as Caleb's ability and willingness to chew and swallow gradually improved over the first days of January.

Caleb's healing process seemed to be boosted by the introduction of solid foods, if ice cream actually fits that category. Bettina observed significant progress, even though she was two provinces away:

Jan 6, 2023 update

The faithful love of the Lord never ends! His mercies never cease. Great is his faithfulness; his mercies begin afresh each morning.

Lamentations 3:22-23

Every day we get to be amazed by something new! So far today I've been able to FaceTime with Caleb three times! He holds the phone now. He nods and shakes his head and waves and gives thumbs up. It's so much fun to talk with him!

Today the speech therapist came to see Caleb. She said that for Caleb to think about moving his facial muscles and forming sounds is like climbing a mountain! This process will take time! But he did follow through with making different mouth shapes and he clearly said "no!"

The speech therapist was pleased that Caleb could say "ah" and "no" in response to her requests. This was a breakthrough. She encouraged Bettina (by phone) to do lots of repetition, and begin with functional words such as "mom," "bye," "yeah," before moving on to greater challenges.

While Bettina, at home in Saskatchewan, was marvelling at Caleb's efforts to communicate, Bruce was breaking new ground with Caleb's diet. Bruce's detailed notebook contains this entry for breakfast on Friday January 6, showing a giant leap forward:

- two yogurts,

- 100 ml. of Ensure,

- three teaspoons of peanut butter = 10 grams = 60 calories

- 1 cup of Moose Tracks

The new lunch routine lower on the same page in Bruce's notes is almost normal:

-two yogurt cups,

-15 grams of peanut butter

-Moose Tracks—1 cup

- apple juice, 50 ml

-cheeseburger—1 bite

The old Caleb could have lived on cheeseburgers and spaghetti; the original Caleb was also known to be a fussy eater, and not a fan of vegetables. Bruce had his work cut out, finding favourites to wake up Caleb's appetite. Helpfully, an aunt brought a batch of home-made spaghetti to tempt her great nephew. The idea didn't take off at first, but gradually, one spoonful at a time, Caleb ate normal meals—punctuated at least three times a day by Moose Tracks.

He was finally reaching his fluid target and was consuming acceptable quantities of calories to promote healing. Vegetables, well, not so much. Bruce was prepared to work on that, too—just not right away.

SECTION FOUR

THE DREAM

CHAPTER TWENTY-THREE

STARTING OVER

aleb's gradual emerging from wherever he had gone was parallel in many respects to what a baby learns in the first year of life. It was as if all the most basic skills had been put on pause and needed to be reactivated.

Babies are born with the ability to swallow and to suck. Caleb could not do this until he became slightly responsive, still only partly awake. However, some innate functions were not yet connected: at the beginning he didn't seem hungry or thirsty. Where was a growing boy's appetite? Or was he just unable to coordinate sucking on a straw and swallowing, at first?

When he finally seemed ready to take in food, he lacked the ability to stay on task. Just as newborn babies suck urgently, and then drift off to sleep when they have hardly consumed anything, Caleb would sit up and seem eager about eating, only to stop and point to his bed.

Over and over, Bruce and Bettina returned to ponder Dr. Ajani's analysis: clearly some of the "wires" were repairing themselves, and some of the "lights" were already on. But many were not. They forced themselves to be patient. Would Caleb eventually be able to eat normally, unassisted? They trusted God that it would happen, but when?

Newborn babies seem to find light shocking or even painful until they adjust. Typically, their eyes squint until the lights are lowered, which is no surprise, since they have come from a dark environment. Caleb opened his eyes infrequently, and never fully, for several days. In case this was partly attributable to light-sensitivity, the care-team produced sunglasses for his activity periods. This prompted some "rock star" comparisons from Bruce and some visitors.

Would he eventually open his eyes fully, and how long might this take?

To the amazement of the hospital staff, Caleb spent only a couple of days in this second infancy. Then he became a tall and gangly toddler, trying to stand, to walk on his own and to express his needs.

Caleb-as-a-toddler quickly found ways to make his wants and intentions known, using techniques more basic than speech. As soon as he could direct the movement of his hands, he would point to the bed when he wanted to end the therapy session. He would point to the bathroom door to show he needed the toilet.

The medical team was impressed and remarked on his speedy progress. He was improving faster than one could turn the pages of a child-development textbook. However, the team members tactfully did not remark on what was missing among his first significant gains: toddlers laugh, cry, and smile. They also verbalize, practicing sounds and generating gibberish, long before anyone can tell what they are trying to say. Not all of Caleb's progress was textbook perfect. When would he reach these missing milestones, if ever? Clearly, in Caleb's damaged, Middle-Earth brain, not all the wires had healed.

His care team would move Caleb to his wheelchair for a feeding session. This was partly observation for the team, partly nutrition for Caleb, and partly a very tiring session that needed to be followed immediately by a nap.

Encouraging him to take the spoon, no matter how messy the result, was another toddler-like stage. He would take the spoon confidently, make a valiant attempt at feeding himself while his nurse held the cup and guided his hand. But too soon he would become exhausted by the effort. He would relinquish the spoon to his nurse. Because he was still hungry, the team member would take over the feeding. At the end of just one small yoghurt cup, he would be too exhausted to continue. He'd stop eating point to the bed.

To his disappointed parent, one of his caregivers repeated, "Remember, this is like climbing a mountain, for him."

CHAPTER TWENTY-FOUR

LIVING THE DREAM

In his toddler-like stage of healing, Caleb's first clear word was "no," again echoing the earliest child-development vocabulary. For Caleb, "no" was a triumph, but he had already been able to indicate preferences by pointing, nodding or shaking his head. "No" did not seem like a huge advance, or even a useful step, at first. However, it was the first little snowball in an avalanche of words.

His ability to speak had been confined to the inside of his head until his mouth and vocal cords could co-ordinate what to do next. Once he started making sounds, he leapt ahead to full sentences within twenty-four hours. He also remembered much more about each day after he began to speak. Clearly, waking and speech were connected in some way.

Most of what Caleb now remembers about his time in the hospital began around January 1. It was piecemeal. When asked a few weeks later to describe his experience from January 1, he said, "I was sure it was a dream."

He explained that the hallmarks of a dream were present: Some of the people were familiar, and behaved in familiar ways. Others were complete strangers, doing odd things to him. Everything looked a bit fuzzy, a bit indistinct, so there was no point in trying to focus, most of the time. No cause for concern: a dream should look dream-like, and will come to an end, he reasoned.

His Dad was nearby, in the dream, but Mom, Eliza, Ethan, and Lukas were far away. He and Dad weren't with the rest. That didn't make any sense, so it had to be a dream. Caleb shared these thoughts with me toward the end of February 2023. He was eager to be interviewed for this book and was still trying to puzzle out what he had experienced.

> *"In the dream, I couldn't talk and could hardly walk. I didn't worry about that, because, after all, it was a dream. While I was in the dream, everything seemed like a game. In the therapy room there were some games that were fun. I thought I should really take advantage of this dream, and all these games, because eventually I'm going to wake up.*
>
> *I made up games to pass the time, too. Some days I didn't want to go to physiotherapy with Charmaine, so I would lie like I was still sleeping, and fake it. They would poke me and shake me. It was a sort of game. Everything seemed like a game.*
>
> *Even eating ice cream was a game, and that was after I had started to talk. I remember the first day I got a bit of ice cream. After supper, Dad was on his phone, and I was in the wheelchair, and had nothing to do. I said to him, twice, to make sure he could hear me, "Ice. Cream." I had only said a couple of words before that, so he was pretty surprised.*
>
> *I made up a game about eating the ice cream, too. I would say to myself, if I get a peanut-butter cup in the next spoonful, I win! That made it even more fun."*

Caleb's ability to remember during the dream-period was inconsistent. There was no sudden waking. Some memories came back to him later, but other "memories" were only prompted by Bettina's notes.

"I remember playing hockey, with Dad and Sarah, but not the first time, with Mom and Mindy. I read about some things in Mom's journal and I don't have any memories of some of it.

I think the earliest thing that I remember about being in the hospital was pulling out the tube. I read about it in Mom's journal. I don't remember pulling it out so many times, but I definitely remember them putting it back in. Or trying to.

I do remember some things that I did with Mom before she went home. We went to the shower room, where you can take a shower while sitting in a chair. Mom gave me the wand to hold. It was a bit weird that I couldn't feel the water, but then, of course, it was a dream."

About a week later, when Caleb was more awake, but still thought he was in a dream, Bruce took him for another shower.

"I was in the shower, and Dad was there, and suddenly I realized I could feel the water. It was warm, and I was getting wet all over. I said to myself, it's still a dream, right? Do people take showers in a dream? I wasn't so sure it actually was a dream, any more."

On January 8, Caleb opened his Christmas presents, with his mother and siblings watching on the phone.

"I remember opening my presents. That was great. I'm not sure if I knew Christmas had happened weeks earlier. I got a big Lego set, and spent a lot of that day building it, start-ing with the helicopter. I remember Mom mentioning that

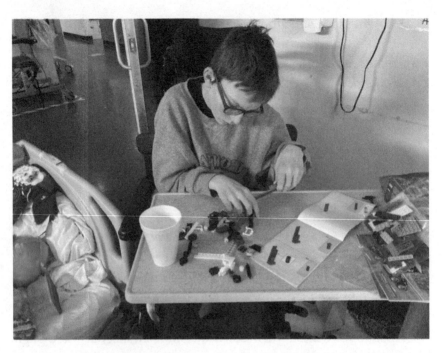

the others, Eliza, Ethan, and Lukas, had already opened their presents from me, and they were excited to see me open the things they had given me. I remember thinking, this dream is very odd. People in this dream know things that people in dreams shouldn't know, like what is going to be in the package that I unwrap. And they have already played with the things I gave them.

Then, on FaceTime, Mom asked me if it was ok that they had gone ahead and worked on the Lord of the Rings jig-saw puzzle. I had been working on it with her and Eliza, and they were continuing. This really struck me as odd: I'm in a dream where other people ask me about things that only I should know about, because it's my dream, and a dream is a completely made-up world, right?

Even so, I was pretty sure it was a dream, because, why would I be in hospital? I wasn't sick. Why would people make me play all these games, ride a tricycle in the hall-way, things like that? In real life those things don't happen.

On one of the days that I was sure it was a dream, I was in the Child Life room and one of the workers asked me to colour a chart, with markers, putting the right colour in the box beside the word "red" and "blue," and so on. I looked at it, and thought it was a colouring exercise for little kids, but I had decided to make the best of these games and activities. I always got praised for how well I was doing, so why not? I didn't think it was very challenging, but I started out very carefully, to impress the Child Life worker. I was staying inside the lines and basically doing a terrific job. I thought.

Several days later, the Child Life worker showed me that paper again. I had made mistakes near the beginning, put-ting colours in the wrong space, then noticing my mistake when the lines and words didn't match up. I was able to stay in the lines, when I started, but only for a while. My colouring got wobbly. By the time I got to the bottom of the page, to the seventh colour, which was black, my colouring looked like a little child scribbling. It was embarrassing to see. I was sure I had aced that assignment!

There were other things that I thought I could do easily, and I would be shocked to find out that I couldn't. Some-times I would find out later that I had improved in some area.

Several days after I was first able to play cards, I noticed my wobbly handwriting when I look at the earlier pages in the scoring book. Dad kept score at first, then he let me do it. I know how to keep score, no problem. But now, when I look at what I did, it's messy, not even in straight columns. In the dream, I thought it was perfect.

I tried over and over to remember what Eliza and I were doing, all in the dream, but before the hospital part of the dream. There was a game, Sam and Frodo, a game Eliza and I play together. I think I remember that, or maybe only because Eliza told me. Then nothing. Then I was stuck in a hospital, for no reason. It was confusing, but all part of the dream, I thought.

In the dream, I could go to sleep, expecting to wake up somewhere else, like home, maybe. But every time, I 'woke up,' I was still in the dream. It got a bit frustrating. I was ready for this dream to be over."

Caleb reflects that he didn't wake up properly until he started talking. Alternatively, he may have started talking because his brain was awake enough to coordinate thoughts, language and vocal cords. There was a definite link between awareness and speech, but which caused the other?

Speech came in stages, and, perhaps, as did waking up. His speech was at first slow, with spaces between the words, followed by exhaustion. Bruce noted that he needed many hours of sleep, in the first days that he regained speech. Truly being awake and having all of his newly repaired circuits firing at once was achieved gradually and was physically draining.

CHAPTER TWENTY-FIVE

SATURDAY JANUARY 7

Back in Stewart Valley, Bettina's new routine involved making herself available by phone whenever Caleb was in bed and wanted Facetime with Mom. This was no easy feat, owing to being in different time zones, having to get Eliza off to school, and to distract Ethan and Lukas long enough to focus on Caleb during the call. Caleb wanted to talk to her two or three times per day, which Bettina was more than willing to do, but sometimes there were a few extra people on the call, as the other children clamored to talk to Caleb.

Bettina and Bruce had discussed the speech therapist's recommendations, and Bettina was eager to get started on simple sounds with Caleb. On Saturday morning, Caleb greeted her with "Hi," and then after a short pause, "Mom." As far as she knew, he had not practiced these words with his therapist. Then, after a bit, he put them together in his first phrase, "Hi, Mom." Bettina felt tears coming.

She did most of the talking on the call, commending him on his efforts, and promising to call back later in the day, after he had rested. They would practice a few more simple, useful words. At the end of the call, Caleb said "Bye." Bettina was amazed.

Caleb wasn't finished with surprises. Later that day, Bettina was on FaceTime again, and asked him what he had for lunch. Referring to the Moose Tracks ice cream, he said a whole phrase at one go, "Peanut butter cups." By this time, Bettina knew that Bruce and Caleb had gone through an entire one-and-a half litre pail of Moose Tracks, so she wasn't really shocked to know that these words were important to her son. But turning to the practicalities of life, she coached him on using his new verbal skills to give simple directions to Bruce or his caregivers. Bettina said, "What would you like to try to say, if you need the toilet?" She offered him options, one-syllable baby-words, such as she would have taught each of her children, when they first began to speak.

Caleb pondered these choices, and said, slowly and deliberately, one word at a time, "I-need-to-go-to-the-bathroom."

"Okay," thought Bettina to herself, "The training wheels are definitely off, and this kid is pedalling on his own."

Sure enough, during the same call, Caleb tried out a few more words and short sentences.

As his endurance and attention span grew, Bettina began to use the FaceTime sessions to read to him from a book that they had read together, before the accident. The book was _Farmer Boy_, a children's historical fiction novel by Laura Ingalls Wilder, who is more famous for _Little House on the Prairie_. Caleb began to ask for a chapter of the book during their FaceTime sessions.

CHAPTER TWENTY-SIX

SUNDAY JANUARY 8

Update for Jan 8, 2023 from Bettina

"Oh, how my soul praises the Lord. How my spirit rejoices in God my Saviour!"

Luke 1:46b-47

Every day we are blown away at how Caleb is progressing!! Now I am having trouble getting anything done at home because Caleb is enjoying FaceTime ☺ this is a good problem to have, ha ha!!

Caleb can ask me to read a chapter in the book we are reading, he asks to see all the different people that are home, and today on FaceTime we got to see him open his Christmas presents!! And he wanted to start building the Lego set from Grandma!! So fun to see!!

Today he worked with Physio on stairs, ate spaghetti for lunch and is asking for me to read more of the book. The one statement he said to me yesterday that went straight to my heart was "Mom, can you bless me?" Wow!! God is good!!

We have so much to be thankful for and we are watching a miracle take place every day!! Please pray for Caleb's strength and stamina to continue getting stronger. He no longer uses a walker. We would say he is awake now and able to stay awake longer so these are amazing improvements.

CHAPTER TWENTY-SEVEN

TUESDAY JANUARY 10

Update for Jan 10, 2023, from Bettina:

"Do not fear, for I have redeemed you;
I have summoned you by name; you are mine.

When you pass through the waters,
I will be with you;
and when you pass through the rivers,
they will not sweep over you.
When you walk through the fire,
you will not be burned;
the flames will not set you ablaze."

Isaiah 43:1b-2

These are the words that Opa—that's what the kids call my father—shared with Caleb today! God will be with you through it all!

In the past two days we have had a different neurosurgeon on the ward, a woman. She and the speech therapist both marvel at how well Caleb is doing. The neurosurgeon said, "Sometimes there is just no medical explanation for how things happen!" (Referring to how quickly Caleb is progressing). In other words, we are seeing a miracle! This neurosurgeon had not seen Caleb before yesterday. She couldn't believe that the initial thought had been that he would need six to twelve months of rehab. Seeing his progress, she thought his time at Bloorview would not be as long as even the six to eight weeks they offer!

And the speech therapist who saw Caleb on Friday and helped him say his first word couldn't believe how well he was already talking by Monday! She used the words "unbelievable" and "impressive"!!

The PT on Saturday was also impressed with Caleb's strength. He took a long walk and then rode the big tricycle all around the hospital "block". She called it his "Turn around day!"

The application to Bloorview Rehabilitation Hospital is submitted. We hope to know in the next week when he will be admitted there. Once he's admitted, I plan to trade spots with Bruce and be with Caleb.

Multiple times a day we are still connecting with Caleb over FaceTime. Today I had a surprise and Bruce showed me a note Caleb had written: Mom I love you and I miss you!

We are so grateful for your continued prayers for Caleb and for being a part of the daily miracles God is granting us!

Reflecting on the new neurosurgeon's remarks, Bruce and Bettina had never contemplated that recovery might require a whole year of rehab. It was a bit sobering to hear the doctor state this opinion, even if it had been eclipsed by Caleb's amazing progress.

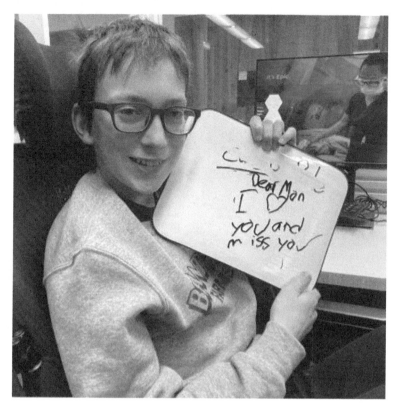

7 Using Facetime, Caleb shows Bettina a message he has written.

CHAPTER TWENTY-EIGHT

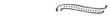

AGITATION, DOUBLE VISION

Not everything about that Tuesday was happy. Caleb returned to a request he had made to Bruce on Monday: when would they be able to go home?

Caleb had heard so many specialists and therapists heaping praise on his progress that he felt empowered. He felt well. He did not feel at all like a person who needed to be in hospital. On Monday night, after asking Bruce when they could go home, Caleb had gone to sleep resolved to wake up "all better."

Caleb:

> "I just decided I had been there, doing nothing, for long enough. In the morning, I was determined I would wake up and be all better. Then we could leave.

The next day, Tuesday, more caregivers, therapists and doctors visited his room and remarked on his amazing progress. This reinforced in Caleb the idea that he really didn't need to be in hospital at all.

> "In the afternoon, I woke up after I had a nap. Just Dad was there. He helped me get into the wheelchair and wanted to feed me dinner. I put up a fuss.

Bruce remembered this landmark day, and not in a good way. It was the first time Caleb has been openly rebellious since regaining consciousness.

"Why am I here? Why do I have to use a wheelchair? I don't need it. I can walk."

True, Caleb had demonstrated his ability to walk in the hospital corridors, assisted by his caregivers, but seemed to be unaware that he was never left alone. The physiotherapist at his elbow was there to guard against falls and any incident that might jar his healing brain. It was also about his balance, endurance and coordination, all of which had a long way to go. Similarly, he was not permitted to climb out of bed or get out of his wheelchair unassisted.

Not accepting Bruce's attempted explanation, Caleb pushed on angrily:

"And why are you feeding me? I can eat. Give me the fork."

Caleb retells this conversation with a touch of chagrin:

Dad didn't know what to do, so he gave me the fork. He had some of Aunt Ann's spaghetti ready to feed to me. It was in pieces so that I could eat it with a fork. I got some on the fork, but almost nothing was on the fork when it got to my mouth. I tried again. Same thing. I was shocked. And pretty disappointed, because maybe there was something wrong with me. Or else I was trapped in the dream, and needed to find a way out.

I asked Dad why I was in a hospital, and he said I had been hit by a car. I didn't think that could be right. Wouldn't I remember? I should have hurt a lot, if I had really been hit, and have bad injuries, but there was nothing like that. But, then, people in dreams say strange things. And even if

I had been in an accident, like Dad said, there was nothing wrong with me now.

"When did that happen?" I asked Dad. I could remember being at Grandma's house, and then nothing. I didn't remember anything about a car accident. He must be wrong.

I was pretty angry. I don't remember it much, but I can see it from Mom's notes. I probably yelled at Dad. He got her on the phone, on FaceTime, right away.

I asked her why I was still in hospital. I told her I was all better now, and wanted to go home. The only thing wrong, I told her, was that I was seeing doubles of things that are far away.

Mom told me, as Dad had, that I was in an accident and hit my head very hard, and had a brain injury.

I was a bit calmer after talking to Mom, but mostly just very tired.

Bettina records this event as the first sign of a stage that is normal in brain-injury patients. She and Bruce had been told to expect outbursts and periods of agitation, perhaps with anger. This phase of Caleb's recovery could last for days, or weeks. It could inhibit his ability to participate in his own rehabilitation, by erasing the cooperative attitude he had exhibited so far. It could also become a permanent, new feature of a patient's personality.

Forewarned of all of this, Caleb's parents braced themselves for a wild ride. But it never came. Aside from the revelation that Caleb had double vision, the storm cloud of agitation, anger and lack of cooperation passed. Certainly Caleb continued to express his wish to go home to Gloryview as soon as possible, but he resigned himself to doing the work of getting better.

With the discussion of continuing his rehabilitation at a different hospital, Caleb was certainly more reluctant to stay in Ontario, and eager to go home. If the choice had been his, he probably would have elected a rehabilitation centre in Saskatchewan or Alberta. Such a plan would only work if they had space available immediately. They did not.

Bruce enlisted the various therapists and specialists to talk to him about what changes they needed to see before he would be ready to go home and to return to school. They tried to make him understand what parts of him were not yet "all better."

One of the neurosurgeons, Dr. Singh, came by to tell them that Caleb's brain signals were not yet normal. Rehab was needed to help the brain get better faster. Despite Caleb's great progress, this was expected to take a few more weeks. Along with Dr. Ajani, Dr. Singh seemed confident that Caleb would make a full recovery, based on his past progress.

The double vision was a surprise, and puzzling to everyone. When had it started? Caleb had unwrapped his Christmas presents two days earlier, played cards, built Lego, climbed stairs, shot pucks into nets, and had written messages to his mom on the white board. Never once had he mentioned double vision. Now, he could be observed reading by following the words with his finger on the page.

Bruce wondered if Caleb was tracing the words with his finger so that he could follow just one line of print, when he was seeing two? Or was it possible that his brain could only read at the speed of a primary schooler, one letter at a time?

The therapists immediately installed a patch over one side of his glasses. This made it easier for him to read, but did not resolve the double-vision problem. For that, they had other methods and exercises. The patch was switched from left to right, and back again, over several days, while the therapists tried different techniques to train Caleb's eyes to work together. It would be several days before the patches could be removed.

CHAPTER TWENTY-NINE

WEDNESDAY JANUARY 11: TRYING TO RECALL EVENTS

The day following Caleb's agitated outburst was the first day he seemed to remember being told about the car accident, although it cannot have been the first time he asked, or anyone mentioned it. He peppered his mother and father with questions about what had happened that day, and what had occurred just before.

"We were supposed to go to Uncle Tom's for dinner. Did we go? I don't remember anything after being at Grandma's."

Gradually, perhaps because Bettina and Bruce told him the story over and over, he "remembered" walking with Eliza in the semi-darkness. Eventually he could rebuild most of the events of that day.

By Thursday, January 12, Caleb's phone calls to Bettina included questions about friends in Stewart Valley, whether his former school would be rebuilt after a fire, whether a neighbour's injured dog was better. He also requested that Bettina buy Ethan a birthday present with Caleb's money, in case Caleb couldn't get home in time for the birthday on January 14.

Bruce notes for January 12: "This afternoon and evening he sounded just like his old self again."

Caleb was still agitating to go home as soon as possible, but he did not show the anger and distress that had marked his outburst on Monday. He had been in hospital for three weeks. He had made enormous and impressive progress from being comatose on arrival, but there was a long way to go.

CHAPTER THIRTY

THURSDAY, JANUARY 12

From Bruce:

John 16:33. "I have told you these things so that you may have peace in me. Here on earth you will have many trials and sorrows. But take heart, because I have overcome the world."

Because of your prayers and God's gracious nature we have experienced His peace and a modern-day miracle. We are grateful and thankful.

Caleb slept a lot yesterday: more than 20 hours! But he was awake enough to beat me in cards. God is knitting the brain's fibres back together. Thank you, Jesus.

We also found out yesterday that the "intake meeting" between the staff at the hospital and the staff at Bloorview Rehab will take place on Tuesday Jan 17. We pray that Caleb can be admitted very soon after that!

CHAPTER THIRTY-ONE

GLORYVIEW

Caleb was homesick almost as soon as he began to regain consciousness. The more phone calls he had with Bettina and his siblings, and the more he regained his communication skills, the stronger was the pull of Stewart Valley and home. What was this place that exercised such a magnetic force on Caleb?

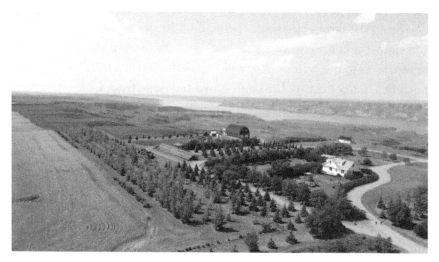

8 Gloryview Farm overlooking Diefenbaker Lake in southern Saskatchewan.

Caleb's home, aptly named "Gloryview," is on the edge of a plateau high above the South Saskatchewan River valley. To the north, the westerly end of Diefenbaker Lake extends from west to east for about twenty kilometres. Beyond the blue of the lake, rolling hills and coulees stretch to forever, fading from grey-green at the shore of the lake to purple in the distance. The panorama is so magnificent that local photographers offer wedding photo-shoots at Gloryview.

Diefenbaker Lake fills the valley once occupied by the South Saskatchewan River. The lake was created in the 1960s, when the Gardiner Dam and the couple River Dam were built. The two dams captured enough water to create a lake more than two hundred and twenty-five kilometres long. A small part of this lake glitters in the prairie sunshine, hundreds of feet below Gloryview.

Bettina's parents, Manfred and Renate Kurschner, known to their grandchildren as Opa and Oma, live in the second floor "loft" of one of the buildings on the farm. Their balcony, closer to the edge of the plateau than the main house, has enough height to provide a view even more breath-taking than the view from the main house. The first floor of this building is a very large room, used as a sports arena by the children, often in good weather but especially in winter.

From the farm's buildings, the land to the north slopes down gently for almost a kilometre of scrub bush and pasture, to the shore of the lake. Closer to the water, out of sight from the top of the hill, neighbours pasture a herd of cattle. The lands down the slope from Gloryview seem park-like. Undulating hills are laced with tractor paths and deer trails. In winter, a tractor trail becomes a toboggan slide for the children.

On the level land of the plateau, farther back from the river valley, Bruce and Bettina's farm consists of cultivated fields. Although they have grain fields, they aren't grain farmers. Instead of farming, the Pates partner with other local volunteers to raise a crop and donate the proceeds to the Canadian Food grains Bank (CFGB), a charity that aims to alleviate hunger worldwide. Neighbours contribute machinery, labour, seeds, fuel, and other inputs required to produce a crop. Bruce Pate has been among the CFGB leaders and volunteers who visit developing economies, working with partner agencies to advance the agricultural skills of individual farmers.

The nearest village is Stewart Valley, where the older Pate children went to school until, tragically, the community's school suffered a devastating fire in 2022. While the Stewart Valley parents and school board struggle with priorities, the children from Gloryview and their friends ride the bus to a school in the village of Waldeck, about twenty kilometres farther away than the school in Stewart Valley.

The Pates have an extensive network of concerned and supportive friends due to a full social life that includes the school parents' association in Stewart Valley and their church in Swift Current. Their local community activities including CFGB plus Bettina's nursing work and Bruce's work with Corteva, an agricultural chemical company, connecting them to many people in the community. Add to this another circle of people who know them through volunteer work and sports, and the result is a great number of people interested in Caleb's recovery.

For Caleb, getting back to normal involved being at Gloryview, getting on the bus to his new school in Waldeck, and being with his sister and brothers. Bettina and Bruce wanted this for him too, but they bowed to the medical advice to take advantage of the high level of care available at McMaster. Everyone shared Caleb's goal of getting back to normal as soon as possible, but Bruce and Bettina knew that the goal line was farther off than Caleb realized.

CHAPTER THIRTY-TWO

FRIDAY JANUARY 14

Jan 14 update, from Bruce:

"The Helper will teach you everything. He will cause you to remember all the things I told you. This Helper is the Holy Spirit whom the Father will send in my name."

John 14:26

God has blessed me with an amazing son. I'm so grateful I get to be Caleb's dad. He is obedient and a great patient. Very polite, always saying please and thank you. His transformation in the last week has been remarkable. He has had to relearn everything and has blown away his medical team in the speed of his recovery. I have heard these comments: "It's been a dream come true for the team to have a patient recover so fast" and also "he is light years ahead of where he was 3 days ago." Yesterday after we built some Lego together, he walked outside with the Physio Therapist, threw a couple of snow balls, walk up a flight of stairs, played some catch and rode the trike around the floor four times without any breaks. His OT played a fun game with him called Hedbanz and she said, "it's wild, the endurance he has now."

Just last Friday morning he did not speak or make a sound and now he is asking great questions, telling stories, remembers a lot and is reading out loud (a little). It was just Wednesday he slept for 20 hours, but for the last two days he has put in 10-12-hour days!

It's been fun to be part of this modern-day miracle.

Thankful for the Spirit of Jesus, His healing touch on Caleb and for everyone's continued prayers.

From Caleb's perspective, the notion that he was still in a dream was fading, but not gone. On Saturday, January 15, he pointedly asked Bruce, "Is this a dream?"

"No."

"Good."

Caleb had asked both Bruce and Bettina to recount the events of the accident day, over and over. He was still struggling with the order of events. He had played in the farm woods. He had gone shopping with Dad for Grandma's Christmas present. Then, in his own word, "nothing." In addition to the gaps, he was still struggling to retain some things he had been told repeatedly while in hospital.

Earlier memories concerning his life in Stewart Valley seemed very clear, and this may have contributed to homesickness. While his previous life was crystal clear, and drew him back to Saskatchewan, he was still trying to bring his lengthy visit to Ontario into focus.

By the mid-January, Caleb left Middle Earth and re-appeared in Hamilton. He didn't arrive there suddenly or dramatically, but gradually he became fully awake, and ceased to ask if he were in a dream. He regained the ability to remember conversations and events from both the previous day and the preceding months. There will probably always be a gap of several days in his memory from December 22 to about January 15.

Having left the coma and the dream behind, he longed to leave Hamilton behind as well, and return to Stewart Valley. That could not happen until more of the work of healing and rehabilitation was complete.

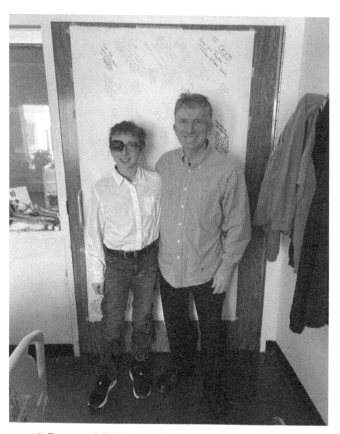

9 On January 15, Bruce and Caleb got a day pass to leave the hospital. They used to opportunity to go to church and have lunch with relatives. Behind them are get-well messages sent from their church in Swift Current, Saskatchewan.

SECTION FIVE:

REHABILITATION

CHAPTER THIRTY-THREE

MONDAY, JANUARY 16

Update from Bruce:

1 Peter 5:10

"And after you have suffered a little while, the God of all grace, who has called you to his eternal glory in Christ Jesus, will restore himself, confirm, strengthen, and establish you."

Caleb has a very good weekend. He is now doing basic life skills on his own: from feeding himself to tying his shoes. We got a leave of absence and went to my cousin's church yesterday, five minutes away. This is the same church Bettina was at with the other children when they lit the candles on Jan 1. The congregation was excited to see Caleb and let him know they were praying for him!

He played some piano, FaceTime'd with some friends back home, and was even asking about homework ☺

Thank you again for praying.

Pray for his double vision to go away, his coordination and reading skills to be restored, and that he would be admitted to Bloorview quickly after tomorrow's intake meeting.

Seeing his interest in the music section of the Child Life room, his worker found sheet music and an electric keyboard that he could keep in his hospital room. Caleb studied music at school. He played drums in a jazz band and euphonium in the junior band at Waldeck school; he knew how to read music. His caregivers were delighted to find another way to engage Caleb's brain, providing him with both an outlet for his growing energy and more ways for his brain to heal.

CHAPTER THIRTY-FOUR

DECIDING TO APPLY TO BLOORVIEW

By Tuesday's team meeting of the McMaster and Bloorview teams, all the pieces had fallen into place for Caleb to continue his rehabilitation in Toronto, at Bloorview. There were options for rehab services a bit closer to home, such as in Saskatoon, but all options involved one parent living in the hospital. The staff at McMaster had sold Bruce and Bettina on the idea that Bloorview was a top-tier facility and they were able to take Caleb right away. In rehabilitation, particularly with young patients, timing is key. To avoid any delay, Bruce and Bettina decided to snatch the opportunity. Somehow, they would cope with living in two provinces and switching places as needed.

For three weeks past the expected end of his Christmas vacation, Bruce's co-workers at Corteva had been covering for him, but they couldn't continue indefinitely. He would have to return to work soon and the family would have to find other ways of caring for Caleb in Toronto and the other children in Gloryview.

CHAPTER THIRTY-FIVE

WEDNESDAY JANUARY 18 — ACCEPTED AT BLOORVIEW

Update for Jan 18, 2023 from Bettina:

"Dear brothers and sisters, when troubles come your way, consider it an opportunity for great joy. For you know that when your faith is tested, your endurance has a chance to grow. So let it grow, for when your endurance is fully developed, you will be perfect and complete, needing nothing."

James 1:2-4

God has been so faithful to us! We are so grateful to all of you for your prayers!

Yesterday we were told that Caleb has been accepted to Bloorview and that he will be admitted on Thursday!! What great news!! He will spend most of Thursday meeting the different members of his therapy team. He will start therapy on Friday.

Bettina will fly to Ontario on Friday and Bruce will fly back to Saskatchewan on Sunday. Please pray for this transition!! We have several people helping with the kids at home this weekend, and please pray that Caleb will have the stamina to keep up with the full, intense therapy schedule. After two weeks of therapy, they will give us a potential discharge date! Our next update will probably be next week ☺

Thank you again for lifting our family up so faithfully!!

On Thursday, the day before Bettina's return to Ontario, Bruce packed up whatever was left in Caleb's room, and they drove to Toronto, to their new temporary home at Bloorview. Caleb got acquainted with his new therapists and got down to work on Friday. Bettina flew in the next day, leaving the children with her parents so that she, Bruce, and Caleb could have a few days alone together.

Update for Jan 23, 2023 from Bettina:

"But they that wait upon the Lord shall renew their strength; they shall mount up with wings as eagles; they shall run, and not be weary; and they shall walk, and not faint."

Isaiah 40:31

Thank you for praying for all the transitions this weekend. Bruce hosted a farewell party in Caleb's room at McMaster last Wednesday afternoon. Staff said the speed of his recovery was remarkable and amazing. They have never had someone recover so much so quickly. They all loved taking care of him!!

Bruce and I enjoyed a lovely weekend with Caleb. We played cards, went for a walk in a nearby ravine, and were able to cook our own meals which Caleb enjoyed. The kids at home enjoyed times with our friends in the day and Oma at night. Bruce arrived safely home on Sunday evening.

This week begins our first full week of therapy and school at Bloorview! Please pray for endurance and strength for Caleb! His double vision is improving, but he still has some blurry vision further away so please pray for complete healing of his sight. We also have a roommate here so that makes nights a bit more interesting. Between my snoring, everyone using the bathroom, nurses checking on us, and alarms going off early, we had an interrupted sleep.

But at 6am, I heard Caleb praying "Lord, thank you that I can have a pass to leave on weekends. Please help Eliza's stuffy nose to get better". He did that all on his own! I smiled in the dark. And then rolled over to sleep some more.

One of the highlights of this week will be going to see the Toronto Maple Leafs play the NY Rangers on Wednesday night, courtesy of a friend!

CHAPTER THIRTY-SIX

THURSDAY JANUARY 26—NHL HOCKEY!

Update for Jan 26, 2023 from Bettina:

"I praise You for I am fearfully and wonderfully made. Wonderful are Your works; my soul knows it very well."

Psalm 139:14

Caleb and I have enjoyed some full days of therapy together! All the therapists are pleased with where he is at when they have been doing their assessments. They have even done harder assessments on him based on how well he has done on the first ones! Every time Caleb tries something a second or third time he has improved. The OT said yesterday, "you're already stronger than Monday! I love how you're planning your moves before you start!" (His executive function)

Caleb remains a joy to be with. We are enjoying reading and playing games in our free time. And he does his fair share of winning ☺ *Last night we braved the "blizzard" and drove to the Leaf's game courtesy of a friend. At one point, Caleb took his eye patch off and said, "Mom I can see better!!" Amazing!! And it was great to see the overtime goal scored right by us by Mitch Marner 19 seconds into OT!! Another bonus was when we left the parkade, the attendant said someone had left a paid ticket so I didn't have to pay! Another miracle!!*

This morning, Caleb was able to have a Google meet with his class in Waldeck! It was great to see everyone and Caleb was able to answer their questions too!

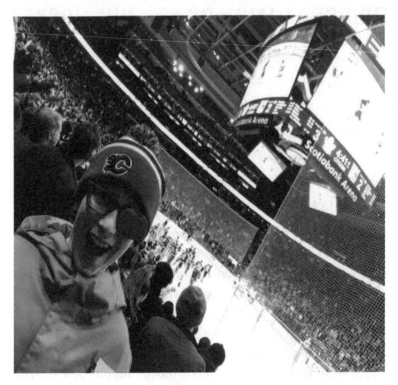

10 At the Scotiabank arena for NHL hockey

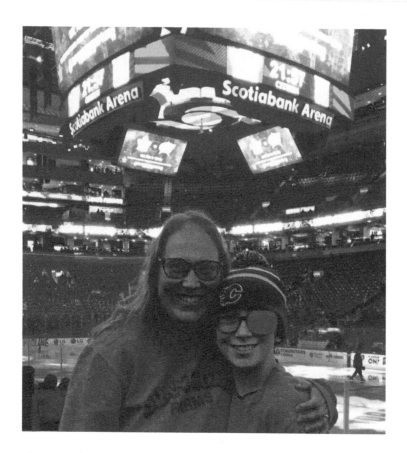

On Tuesday Jan 31 at 11:15 we will have a family meeting with the team to discuss their plans for Caleb as well as a potential discharge date!! We will send another update after that.

This weekend we will use our weekend pass to visit family in Brantford so we are looking forward to that! Sleep has been improved here since the first night (thanks for praying!) but we still look forward to sleeping in a real bed ☺

Please continue to pray for full restoration of Caleb's vision and for the fine tuning of coordination and memory and strength. He's handling the long days fairly well so we are grateful 🙏

CHAPTER THIRTY-SEVEN

TUESDAY, JANUARY 31 — CALEB GETS COVID

Update for Jan 31, 2023

"Jesus looked at them intently and said, 'Humanly speaking, it is impossible. But with God everything is possible.'"

We have definitely had a front-row seat to watching God do the impossible this past month!! We are also very grateful for your continued prayers and support! We can feel it!!

And then some things happen or come along that don't make sense but we still need to be thankful! On Monday, at our first therapy session, Caleb was more tired and also showed a bit of a runny nose. I thought he just had a busy weekend and needed a bit more rest. When we let the nurse know, that began a series of decisions that were kind of out of our hands. Caleb was swabbed and we were asked to go home and self-isolate until he was 24-hour symptom free.

But then last night they called to say his swab shows he has Covid! Surprise! Now we get to isolate for 10 days!

"Go home" does not mean Stewart Valley, sadly. It means we will live at Tom and Dawn's farm, and keep Caleb away from Grandma and everyone else until we can return to Bloorview.

But we still have much to be thankful for: we each have a quiet and peaceful bedroom with a real bed to sleep in, a beautiful farm to get outside on, and great family to support us. And Caleb is already feeling better—after a 12-hour sleep!

Our first day back to on-site therapy will be Feb 13th since our technical first day back after isolating was supposed to be Feb 10 and that's a Friday.

So Caleb's new tentative discharge date is now March 2. We will diligently work on therapy from home and hopefully they will see much improvement in Caleb by Feb 13!!

We can't always know why things happen the way they do but we are grateful that we know God is in control and has His reasons!!

Please keep our family in prayer as the separation is not the easiest thing. For now we are all coping well, but we have another month to go. And Caleb continues with double vision. We have exercises to work on that so we hope that will improve soon as well. Thank you!

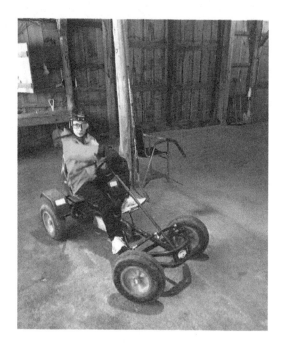

11 Rehab continues in a barn at Brantwood Farm.

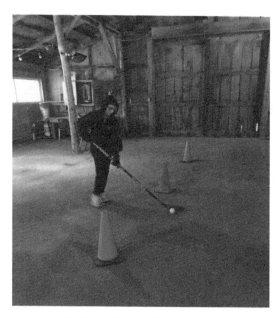

12 Puck handling drills at Brantwood.

Things were going well with remote therapy and remote learning at Brantwood Farm until about eight days into Caleb's period of COVID self-isolation. He had not yet tested negative for COVID when Bettina began to get symptoms. Sure enough, the COVID virus had found her. Time to figure out what was next.

Then Bruce's brother Jim came up with a new solution: Heather and Jim Pate had a vacation house in the beautiful village of Niagara-on-the-Lake. Heather and Jim didn't use it much in winter. It was furnished and ready to turn the key and walk in. Bettina and Caleb moved in on February 3 and resumed their self-isolation, remote learning and remote therapy. It was a little lonelier than living at Dawn's and Tom's, but safer for others.

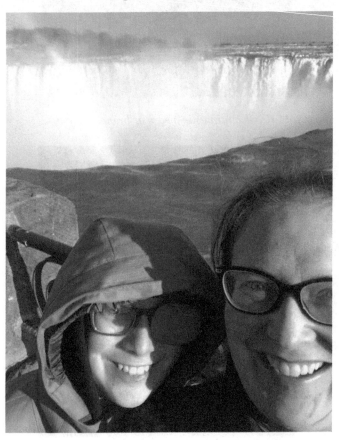

13 A beautiful February day at Niagara Falls.

When Caleb's day's work was done, they played cards and other games, built Lego and even watched TV—a rare indulgence in Bruce and Bettina's family. Finally, on February 8, Bettina's COVID test was negative. She and Caleb celebrated by enjoying a day of being tourists. They visited world-famous Niagara Falls and the tourist area surrounding it, and inspected one of the area's historic forts, both only a short drive from Niagara-on-the-Lake.

By the time the novelty of having their own home in Niagara-on-the-Lake had worn off, it was time to return to Bloorview. When they got there, Bettina took advantage of her weekly check-in with the social worker to discuss a possible early discharge for Caleb, who was upset about having missed Ethan's birthday and his Oma's. It appeared that he would also miss Eliza's, on February 20. Homesickness was taking its toll.

CHAPTER THIRTY-EIGHT

MONDAY FEBRUARY 13 —BACK TO BLOORVIEW

With isolation finally over, Bettina and Caleb resumed in-person school and therapy classes at Bloorview.

They expected that he would have three full weeks of therapy before the projected discharge date of March 2. Bruce booked a flight to return to Ontario on Saturday, February 18. Bettina flew back to Saskatchewan on the following day.

On Monday, February 20, Bruce remarked to the staff at Bloorview that the therapy schedule seemed pretty light, compared with previous weeks. In response, the staff gave him the news that Caleb's discharge date had been advanced to Friday, February 24. There were only four days of therapy left!

Caleb was over the moon with this news. He beamed as he spoke to his mother and siblings via FaceTime. Bruce had scarcely adjusted to the change of time zones, and it was time to make more travel arrangements.

Bruce and Caleb worked hard for the last four days of therapy. Then it was time to pack up and head to Brantford. After a brief overnight visit with family there, they were off to the Toronto airport to start their journey back to Gloryview.

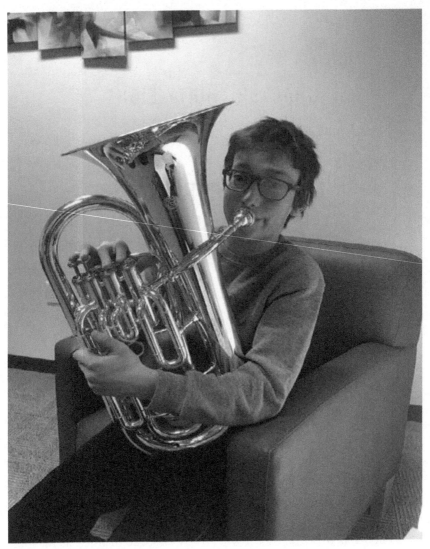

14 Music class in the "school" at Bloorview Children's Hospital.

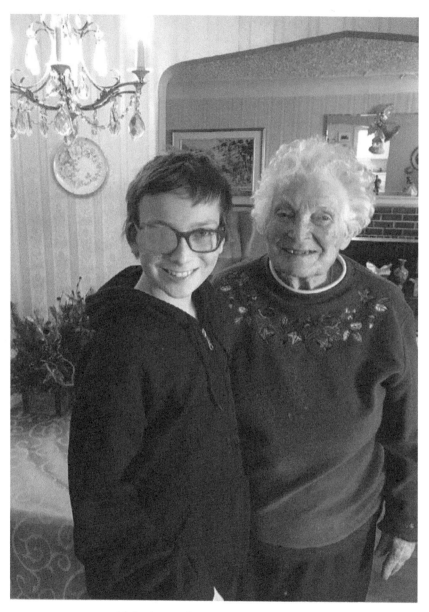

15 Saying good-bye to Grandma Doreen.

CHAPTER THIRTY-NINE

SATURDAY TO SUNDAY, FEBRUARY 25 AND 26

Saturday was probably the longest, most gruelling day of those that Caleb could remember, made more agonizing by his eagerness to be home. They began the day at Brantwood, said their goodbyes, travelled more than an hour to get to the Toronto airport, and waited over an hour to board. Then they waited another hour on the plane. The hours of evening were slipping away. They would fly across two time zones in the dark, arriving well after midnight, Saskatchewan time.

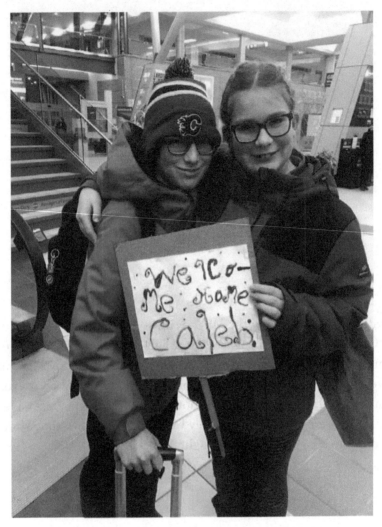

16 Eliza greets Caleb at the airport in Regina.

Bettina's trip to the Regina airport was one hour shorter than Bruce and Caleb's three-an-a-half-hour flight. She and Eliza did not leave home until Bruce's and Caleb's flight was on the way.

When the weary travellers eventually straggled out into the airport lounge for some serious hugs, the clock was creeping toward 2 a.m.

They all set out for Gloryview with two children who were beyond tired. Caleb and Eliza slept in the back seat. They drove into their farm lane, at long last, arriving at 4 a.m.

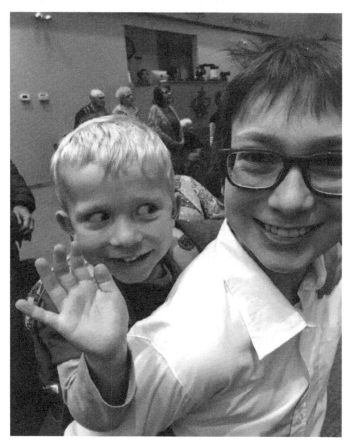

17 Lukas celebrates Caleb's first Sunday back at Trailview Alliance Church.

The time to get caught up on sleep was brutally short. They made it to church in Swift Current after about four hours of shut-eye, probably a little less due to the excitement of the day. There they met Bettina's parents who brought Ethan and Lukas with them. Everyone was over-joyed to see a slightly exhausted but grinning Caleb.

The congregation at Trailview Alliance Church in Swift Current was thrilled to have Caleb and his family back. Bruce and Bettina thanked the congregation and pastor for all of their support, messages and prayers. Caleb was given an opportunity to speak to the congregation, as well. He talked about learning to trust God in Jesus, through his journey back to health.

SECTION SIX

PRAIRIE ROADS

CHAPTER FORTY

CORRECTION LINES

Prairie roads are famously straight. Survey crews attempted to impose a flawless grid on Earth's surface, with only right-angle intersections. This seemingly-perfect geometry only works to a point. Unavoidably, rivers and gullies introduce curves, dips and steep hills. In addition, the curvature of the planet requires the insertion of correction lines into an otherwise-orderly scheme.

Re-entry to home and school life was mostly smooth for Caleb and his family, but not entirely. There were bumps, gullies, and corrections as there are in the roads of southern Saskatchewan.

On Monday morning, February 27, Caleb was back at school in his regular class in Waldeck, Saskatchewan, having missed about seven weeks of regular instruction. During his absence he had fought back from the loss of consciousness, of speech, of memory, of mobility and coordination and he even had to re-learn how to eat. A person older than Caleb with a similar injury might have been on the sidelines for many months, perhaps up to a year, but Caleb was ready to jump right back into the game. Or he thought he was.

At school, it wasn't the actual academic work that challenged Caleb, it was the re-discovery of being one in a class of many. Both at McMaster and at Bloorview he had been the only pupil in his class and he had enjoyed star-treatment. Now his brain was adjusting to working in groups, waiting his turn to ask a question, and striving with others for the teacher's approval. He might have enjoyed an hour or two of celebrity status upon arrival at school, due to the fact that everyone for miles around knew about his accident and his hospitalization in Ontario. By about noon on the first day, with Caleb back in his old desk, and looking just as he had before; the gloss wore off, and it was business as usual.

Bettina had discussed Caleb's return to school with the teachers at Waldeck Elementary School. She had transported homework materials from Saskatchewan to Bloorview in the third week of January, when she and Bruce swapped places. She also kept Caleb on top of his homework when they were unexpectedly required to self-isolate, far from the tutors at Bloorview. By the end of his period of private tutoring, Caleb was approximately where his classmates were, in math. His reading skills were close to the speed and comprehension that he needed, but not there yet. Keeping up in a class with distractions would be a struggle.

In early January, Caleb's first attempts at speech had been flat and mechanical-sounding, without modulation. By the time he rejoined his classmates at Waldeck Elementary School, he had vastly improved. He did not betray anything the therapists would call "deficits."

Because he looked and sounded just the same as he had at the end of 2022, his classmates treated him just as they always had. This was both good and bad. No child wants to be singled out in an embarrassing way, but there were some areas where he needed, and got, special attention.

In a classroom with groups working at different levels, the prospect of being able to advance to the next group can be a motivator or a source of frustration. It was both, for Caleb, as he readjusted. During his nearly two-month absence, he had missed some of the Waldeck school's units of social studies and geography. His teachers allowed these to slide.

Caleb had always been a diligent student, and that had not changed, but he did experience more exhaustion. The therapists at McMaster and Bloorview had commented that while his brain had successfully re-mapped itself for mental activities, the endurance for doing the tasks for long periods would take longer to rebuild. When he reached his limits, the exhaustion in his brain could trigger irritation, which was not characteristic of Caleb. Bettina noticed this at home, and assumed it might be evident at school, on occasion.

Music class proved to be the biggest challenge for his endurance.

The music teacher for several rural schools in their area visited each school once a week. There were not enough music students to form a band unless they all came to the same location, Irwin Elementary School in Swift Current, for band practice on Thursdays. So Bettina would drive Caleb to Swift Current, a half-hour drive from home.

Driving Caleb to Swift Current and picking him up was less tiring for him than the routine hour-long school bus ride to Waldeck on regular school days. Waldeck is only a half-hour away from Gloryview Farm by car, but the circuitous school bus route takes an hour. Getting up early and spending a big chunk of the day on a bus is routine for school children in rural areas.

At three o'clock on Thursdays in Swift Current Caleb played drums for the jazz band for over an hour. Afterwards, he played his euphonium in the junior band until six o'clock. Thus, for jazz band, he would focus on reading music, counting, watching the leader, listening to his bandmates, while keeping his hands and feet moving for the drum sticks and pedals. Then, moving from percussion to brass for junior band, he needed to form the embouchure with his lips, breathe deeply and blow with the correct pressure, timing and fingering. Band practices provided a very thorough way to overheat his recently repaired brain circuits.

Toward the end of his first day back in the organized chaos of band class, Caleb's music teacher noticed something she would previously have thought impossible. As the clock ticked up toward six o'clock, she finished with the woodwinds and asked them to pack up quietly while the brass section had a last run-through of a difficult part. Turning toward the brass players, she saw the euphonium was lying on the floor beside Caleb's chair. He had slumped forward, head hanging over his knees, and appeared to be sleeping. The cacophony of band class was still bashing, buzzing, and tooting around him, but Caleb's brain simply shut it all out. He was done.

The teacher briefly considered whether Caleb was in some sort of crisis rather than just asleep. Getting to him, past music stands, book-bags and student legs, was not easy. The other students had just begun to notice their sleeping classmate and registered surprise and amusement.

Just at that moment, she saw Caleb's mother peering through the classroom, ready to drive Caleb home. She caught Bettina's eye and beckoned her to enter the room.

While the other students were chatting to each other and pack-ing up to go home, a few were pointing at Caleb and giggling. Bettina reached Caleb, still folded over in his chair, and so sound asleep that she had to shake him. Groggily, he sat up, gave her a big hug and asked, "Mom, why is it so noisy?"

When Bettina and the teacher realized how draining the three-hour band practices were for Caleb, they arranged for him to have a rest, snack and break, in between jazz and junior band. Bettina also got approval to keep him home from school on Thursday mornings, so that he could conserve his energy for band practice sessions in the afternoon.

Caleb's parents chose not to take him out of music class. The sense of exhilaration from actually mastering and performing a piece of music is one of the best natural highs a child can have. When children per-form music as a group, and hear the applause of an audience, they have a shared sense of pride and accomplishment. As a group, they and their teacher may experience a rush of joy and relief bordering on giddiness when they get to the last note on the last page, more or less at the same time.

Teachers see the happiness that music creates. Success begets suc-cess, and joy begets joy, and makes all the agony of practicing worthwhile. It overcomes all the pain of hearing more than a dozen instruments, some slightly out of tune, playing wrong notes together, while learning a song. Despite these sacrifices to their eardrums, music teachers throw themselves into this work, and many find it hard to retire!

With this in mind, Bruce and Bettina wanted to keep music in Caleb's school life.

Bettina's eldest son, Micah, holds down a regular job in Swift Current, but makes music his consuming hobby, and plays several instruments. He would love to devote all his energies to his music. Bettina envisions Caleb following in Micah's footsteps. Even if he doesn't, music will enrich his recovery and, probably, the rest of his life.

CHAPTER FORTY-ONE

ATHLETICS

Other subjects at school may not have been as thoroughly draining as band class, but there were challenges in other ways. Gym class requires a balancing of challenges and risks for all students, but particularly for Caleb.

Team sports, such as basketball, typically are taught by pitting one half of the class against the other, but Caleb needed to avoid being accidentally or deliberately knocked to the ground. For him, basketball practice was restricted to competing one-on-one with a classmate and trying to sink shots. This was better than shooting hoops all alone, but not remotely as exciting as taking a pass, dribbling the ball down the court, and making the shot.

Until recently, the barn at Gloryview Farm was Caleb's arena for roller-blade hockey with his school friends and sometimes his dad, in all seasons. Christmas of 2022 changed that: now, when his friends come over, everyone wears running shoes for floor-hockey. This slows down the game, but reduces the risk that Caleb might take a body-check and land on the hard floor. At least he is still allowed to play, but not at the accelerated speeds achievable on roller-blades. Predictably, Caleb races through his after-dinner clear-up chores and agitates for ball hockey in the barn almost every evening.

"I'm done, Dad, c'mon, let's go. It's ball hockey time. Dad, c'mon!"

Bruce remembers the advice he was given, on Caleb's discharge from Bloorview: "Just go and live your life." Bruce has followed that advice, but he views the fragility of children's bodies through new lenses. So, no roller-blades for now. And no ice-hockey, for now. Hockey, both played and watched, has long been Bruce's passion, as well as Caleb's. Leaving contact sports at least for a time is disappointing, but a necessary adjustment.

CHAPTER FORTY-TWO

FAMILY LIFE

Caleb spent nearly two months, after coming out of his dream, with the focused attention of one parent or the other. Some of that time was shared with a team of professionals: therapists, doctors, nurses, and others. These people were also his cheerleading squad, hailing every gain that he made and marveling at the speed of his progress. That much daily adulation is uncommon in life and could not be sustained once he was back home. Expectations there were much more mundane: keeping his room tidy, taking his turn with dishes, doing homework on his own, clearing the snow with the garden tractor. There was appreciation, but no lavish praise, because these were his normal activities.

Due to the COVID-19 pandemic, part of Caleb's early recovery was spent in self-isolation with just Bettina, first in Brantford and then in Niagara-on-the-Lake. Bettina supervised his physical exercises, and made sure he had telephone contact with some of his therapists, especially the speech therapist, but there was a lot of time to relax and just spend time together. Caleb had enjoyed having his mother all to himself. Bettina remembered that period warmly, too, but, once they were all together again at the farm, she didn't have time to think much about it. The whirlwind of family life in Stewart Valley had resumed.

After everything Caleb had experienced in sixty days, from the praise of his care team to the exclusive attention of his parents, as if he were an only child, a smooth re-entry to daily family life would have been astonishing. It wasn't smooth, of course.

Sibling time was one of the hardest aspects of re-entry, and the one that surprised his parents the most. Caleb was very attached to his siblings but had not exercised the part of his brain that needed to adjust to having them around all the time. For two months, he had played cards with adults, built Lego with adults, played floor hockey with adults, and so on. He had seen other children, but they were hospital patients, also in recovery. At home, Ethan and Lukas were always getting into his things, just as they had before, but his ability to cope with them was seriously diminished. He had to re-learn not to snarl when they got too close to his Lego sets.

Managing irritations between siblings is nothing new for Bettina and Bruce. The unknown element is wondering which verbal dust-ups are related to injured or exhausted brain circuits, and which are just normal family dynamics, as their son stretches up toward adolescence. They know that a teenager will choose life's roads based on his own interests and passions, sometimes against parental advice. Those roads will almost certainly have ruts, bumps and washouts. The teen will learn to cope. They wonder if Caleb's brain injury will make his road more difficult, but they cannot know. Not yet.

CHAPTER FORTY-THREE

ELIZA

Eliza, too, was delighted to have Caleb home, but there were consequences. She had to relinquish her temporary position as the oldest-child and helper-of-parents.

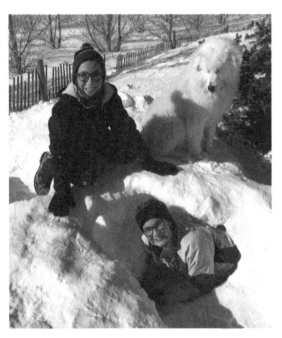

18 Caleb, Eliza and Bear building a snow fort.

She also had to slip back into the younger-sister role, in which Caleb sometimes treated her as a close friend, but was just as likely to exclude her when his school friends came over to play. She was an understudy again, a familiar role: always Sam, never Frodo. Not everything about having Caleb home was as perfect as she had imagined, when she could only see him for a few minutes each day on the phone.

Eliza was also unable to shake her memories from that horrendous December. Her Grandma Doreen stated that 2022 would remain in her memory as the Worst Christmas of All Time. Eliza shared that feeling.

One day in the school cafeteria, while Caleb was still in Ontario, she had a flashback. Eliza let her mind wander. She was half-listening to school mates whose Christmas adventures seemed trite in comparison to hers. Suddenly, she could sense pulsing blue and red lights all around her. She felt paralyzed with fear, just as if she were back at the edge of Powerline Road. She must have had a glazed look, or perhaps she had disengaged from the group for long enough to catch their attention.

"Hey, 'Liza, are you okay?" someone asked.

She lurched back into the present, and waved them off, so that her schoolmates wouldn't pursue the matter. But in that moment, she had not been okay. Those lights, those fearful moments, the recollection of how limp and heavy Caleb was when she tried to drag him, and how his eyelids fluttered; it had all come flooding back. She remembered her panic, mixed with anger, when he wouldn't answer her, or couldn't answer her. She remembered the driver's surly tone, "Dude, what were you thinking?"

How long would these scenes keep replaying in her mind, unwanted and frightening?

Bettina and Bruce are aware that Eliza still carries something akin to post-traumatic stress. Her mental healing, with the help of her parents and professional counsellors, may take as long, or longer, than Caleb's. He does not have any memory of that dark evening with its throbbing red and blue lights. For Eliza, the memories are real and very vivid.

When Eliza first returned to school, she was shocked when on entering the school gym, the school colours—red and blue—on banners on the walls brought back the memory of pulsating ambulance lights. Bruce and Bettina have been involved in planning for rebuilding the Stewart Valley school. Eliza is looking forward to the re-built school, to get away from her blue and red world at Waldeck.

Eliza also struggled to express her angst over Caleb's return to Saskatchewan. Shortly after Caleb had returned to Stewart Valley and resumed attending school, Eliza confided to her mom that her friends just didn't understand how much the incident had affected her. In February she tried to tell her school friends that it was as if Caleb had died on the day of the accident, and so had she. Her friends laughed at this notion, saying, "That's just silly! Caleb was here yesterday! You're here today. Nobody's dead."

But Eliza saw it differently: there was something about her brother, her best friend, that was broken, missing, perhaps gone forever. Eliza was shaken by her realization that the Caleb who came back from the rehab hospital in Ontario wasn't the same brother who played Sam-and-Frodo with her on December 22, 2022. The 2023 version of Caleb looked the same but something inside had changed. He had angry outbursts, was rough with her, had no patience with his little brothers or her. She could no longer feel close to him, could no longer trust him with her private thoughts and ideas. She felt the loss deeply.

After one particularly stinging disagreement, Eliza protested that Caleb should be more grateful to her. She was still haunted by the chilling minutes after the accident happened, when she had dragged him off the road, away from what she feared would be a possibly worse catastrophe, being hit twice.

"I saved your life," she exclaimed.

"The doctors saved my life," Caleb replied, and turned on his heel.

Initially, upon arriving home from Ontario, Eliza had declined any therapy. However, with Eliza's revelation about how memories of December 22 still haunted her, Bruce and Bettina set up regular counselling. Bettina was unsure how Eliza would respond to this news, so she broke it to her while they were in the car together. Bettina finds this strategy useful for sensitive topics: one-to-one, privacy, and no eye contact. To her amazement, Eliza expressed no resistance this time. Instead, she was grateful.

"Thanks, Mom, I was sort of hoping you would."

Meanwhile, Bruce and Bettina watched Caleb's changed behaviour closely. They managed his bedtime as if he were a much younger child. They separated him from the others in the evenings and this helped to prevent blow-ups.

CHAPTER FORTY-FOUR

SUMMER

The Pate Family makes two annual trips to Ontario. In addition to their Christmas trip, they come in the summer, to visit family and spend time at the family cottage on a small lake near Bancroft, Ontario.

To his grandmother and all family members at the cottage that summer after the accident, Caleb appeared to be in top form. He improved his water-ski skills, and enjoyed wake boarding and knee-boarding, as well as swimming. He also slept ten hours a day. His parents weren't sure whether to attribute this to being on the threshold of his teen years or his still-healing brain.

While his physical progress gave her no concerns, Bettina reflected that in the psycho-social realm, it was as if Caleb needed to re-focus. He needed to re-learn to read the signals around him, those cues from parents and peers about what behaviour is acceptable.

The family was accustomed to spending a few minutes after the evening meal for family devotions, usually a Bible reading and reflection or questions on the topic, but Caleb-in-recovery was too flippant and disruptive for this to work. After several unsatisfactory attempts to get him to observe some boundaries on his humorous interruptions, Bettina instead introduced a different routine: individualized devotional time with each child in their own rooms at bedtime.

Gradual, over the months of spring and summer, Caleb became less combative with his siblings, and even won back Eliza's trust. As more time passed, it became harder to distinguish effects of the trauma from the changes wrought by growth spurts and hormones.

In September his teacher commented to Bettina that he was cutting up in class, and needed to work on more appropriate behaviour. However, by November, the same teacher confirmed that these issued had resolved: Caleb was re-learning appropriate boundaries, and reining in his exuberant class-clown tendencies. Invisibly, healing was still happening.

CHAPTER FORTY-FIVE

SHAUNAVON

In the fall of 2023, Caleb's counsellor in the Acquired Brain Injury Outreach team invited Bettina and Caleb to speak to at an event for students in Grades 10, 11 and 12 at the high school in Shaunavon, Saskatchewan, about two hours from their home in Stewart Valley. The event, organized annually by the school board in cooperation with the police and health services, is aimed at preventing alcohol-related brain trauma in youth. Caleb and Bettina accepted the challenge and began to plan their shared presentation. Bettina would have a large part, as she had been able to make many observations long before Caleb could.

There was a packed schedule for the day. The program included enacting a mock accident scene with real-life first responders and students as "victim" actors. There was also an exercise for students to try to conduct normal activities such as eating lunch while encumbered with a "disability" such as being in a wheelchair, or unable to see, or to have their hands restrained to simulate paralysis. Caleb didn't have to use much imagination to go back in his mind to the day when he could hold a fork, but could not get food to his mouth.

Bettina thought the program that day was excellent, and she was happy to have the opportunity to share Caleb's experience in Shaunavon. Nonetheless, she has two regrets about that day. The first was about the scheduling of their presentation. They were the last item in the busy program. That was deliberate, because having a local boy with lived experience of a serious injury made them the feature attraction, the "big finish" for the day. Still, the timing was tough on Caleb. He wasn't fresh, and he was also deeply troubled by one of the previous presentations, a film.

Bettina's second regret is that she did not know the content of a road-safety film that the police normally in the afternoon part of the program. If she had known, she would have found some way to prevent Caleb from seeing it. The short film was a dramatic re-enactment of a traffic accident, intended to impress on the students how much can change in an instant. The film shows a seemingly normal street scene, and then, as if out of nowhere, there is a careening car, a crunch, a simulation of a flying body, screams and then a scramble of by-standers and first responders.

Although the circumstances of the re-enactment were nothing like what had happened to Caleb, it affected him deeply. For months he had been frustrated with having no memory of the moments before his accident, nor of what it felt like to be hit, or to fall onto the pavement. He thought he should have a memory of this. And of course his injured brain stored no memories of what Eliza had clearly seen and heard in the aftermath. This allowed him to treat the whole "car accident story" as a dream or a fiction, when he first became alert enough to ask why he was in hospital.

Then, suddenly and unexpectedly, in the darkened arena where the event was held, the huge projection screen showed what could have been his own missing memories: a skid, a crunch, a body landing, a chilling silence, then sirens, police, ambulances, firetrucks, stretchers. Caleb, sitting beside Bettina, was still and silent for several minutes. If he could have withdrawn into a shell like a turtle, he would have. Bettina wasn't at all sure he would be able to do their presentation later that afternoon.

At the appointed time, Caleb managed to carry on, but to Bettina he seemed to lack his normal sparkle. In hindsight, she wishes they had skipped the film and saved Caleb from that part of an otherwise excellent day.

Their presentation included examples of physical skills and abilities that needed to be gradually re-learned. Bettina emphasized how a large team of specialized caregivers helped with this process, and how fortunate Caleb was to be able to make a full recovery.

Bettina hopes that their contribution gave the students at Shaunavon a heightened awareness of the fragility of their own bodies and minds.

CHAPTER FORTY-SIX

CHRISTMAS 2023 IN BRANTFORD

As the year-end approached, Bruce booked the family's flights to Toronto. Once again, they would bunk in at his mother's house on Powerline Road for a couple of nights, visit all of his brothers and their families, then drive to the cottage. There, Bruce and Bettina would sit by the fire while the kids got the winter holiday that had been derailed in 2022.

Eliza was a little anxious about whether the anniversary date would bring more bad luck, so Bruce and Bettina were determined to help everyone have a normal day and celebrate the opportunity to visit family once again.

December 22 came and went. Christmas followed soon after. There were crowded meals at Tom and Dawn's and the homes of other relatives, Christmas carols at church, new toys and inevitably lots more Lego for Caleb. The Worst Christmas Ever was fading into memory, even for Grandma Doreen.

Of all the hugs and smiles that greeted Caleb at family events in Brantford, none was warmer than that of ER nurse Brooke Newsome. Busy with her nursing career and planning her wedding with Andrew Pate for the summer of 2024, Brooke had not thought much about her second-to-last shift before Christmas in 2022. While hugging Caleb, it all came back. It has crossed her mind that night, one year earlier, that he might not make it to see the New Year. Now she worried that she might burst into tears, so she stepped back and teased him about the Calgary hockey team instead.

Being back in Brantford made Bettina think again of the driver. Surely the events of December 22, 2022 must have changed his Christmas as well as theirs. During the year, she had tried on two occasions to pass a message to him through the Brantford police services. She realized this wasn't their priority, and wasn't surprised to get no reply. Nonetheless, she hoped the police had informed the driver that Caleb was fine, was back at school, and had resumed the life of a normal pre-teen, one obsessed with Lego, the Calgary Flames, ball-hockey and Moose Tracks ice-cream.

CHAPTER FORTY-SEVEN

LOOKING AHEAD

The brain itself is a miracle: it learns, it stores memories, it motivates, it hopes and dreams. It generates emotions.

The recovery of a young person's brain from a severe injury, such as Caleb suffered, is another miracle, involving the extraordinary ability of a child's brain to regenerate and restore. A doctor commenting on Caleb's recovery remarked that a young person's brain is able to rebuild neural pathways much faster than an adult brain with a similar injury. Being eleven at the time of the incident was Caleb's winning ticket.

For the most part, Caleb's amazing recovery process happened while he slept. It happened out of anyone's view, and largely unassisted by medical experts. For medication, he had about sixteen hours of sedation, followed by a saline drip to help decrease swelling, and Tylenol for a few days when it was not clear whether he was in pain. Other medical steps were limited to a feeding tube and a breathing tube, each for only a few days. There were no surgeries or other invasive steps. Being with Caleb, as Bettina and Bruce remarked, gave a close-up view of a miracle slowly unfolding.

Did the constant presence of family members by Caleb's bedside speed his recovery? Was Caleb even aware of a steady rotation of parents and other caring relatives, over the first few days? What part did prayer play in his recovery, either those prayers that he consciously heard, or those hundreds voiced in places far away from McMaster hospital?

Caleb was discharged from Bloorview ready to return to life as a Grade Seven student. In terms of the illustration favoured by Dr. Ajani, Caleb's brain wiring was repaired and all the lights were working. His recovery met Dr. Ajani's expectations, but the speed at which healing took place was startling, even to the team members at McMaster.

Dr. Ajani's model does not have a place for the other functions that happen inside the brain: emotions, imagination, conscience, curiosity, to name a few, and yes, even dreams. The brain is the home of the body's guidance systems of temperament, personality, moods and so on. These systems, out of sight and out of reach, are tricky to tune up. Caleb may need to re-calibrate from time to time.

To have a calamity of this nature occur practically on the doorstep of a renowned children's hospital was of great benefit. Bettina, having worked in a modest-sized hospital in rural Saskatchewan for many years, was awed by the level of care, resources, and expertise available at McMaster—and not only for Caleb, but for his family as well.

The team of professionals who work with children, both at McMaster and Bloorview, see the most severely sick and injured children in Ontario. For professional survival, they learn to temper their expectations. Knowing this, Bruce and Bettina were gratified to read genuine astonishment and delight on the faces of Caleb's care team, as he progressed day by day. Not every sick or injured child will be wakeboarding or water-skiing six months later: his parents know this, and are immensely grateful to God, as well as to the medical teams.

Upon their return to Saskatchewan, they continued to be supported by an excellent network of follow-up care for brain-injury patients and families. All of these supports made the return to "normal life" smoother for everyone.

Bruce and Bettina would add that the outcome reflects the strong support of church, family and community to help the entire family get to this point.

Although this is the last page, this story isn't over. Caleb and his family are living the sequel now. Perhaps they will write Part Two in the future.

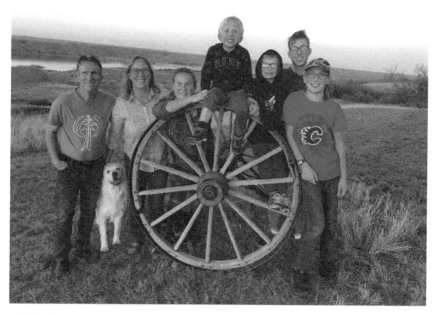

19 The Pates in 2023: Bruce, Bettina with Bear, Eliza, Lukas, Ethan, Micah, Caleb.

HOW THIS BOOK HAPPENED

As a first cousin to Bruce, I was among those who were notified of Caleb's injuries within an hour of the event on December 22, 2022. I live in Dundas, Ontario, which is a community on the highway that Caleb's ambulance used to get to McMaster Hospital.

My husband, Rev. Jim Cairney, is the pastor referred to in the early chapters. He arrived at the hospital not far behind the ambulance. He stayed with Bruce and Bettina until Caleb was stabilized then transferred to Pediatric Intensive Care (PICU).

Both Jim and I were part of the group of relatives who took shifts staying with Caleb, even for overnights, so that Bruce and Bettina could have time with the other children. After Bettina returned to Saskatchewan in early January, we were among those who took afternoon shifts with Caleb so that Bruce could slip away from the hospital and have dinner with his mother in Brantford. It was our privilege to be in the room to witness some of Caleb's milestones, and to celebrate with his family and, in my case, to be taught the rules of Shanghai Rummy by a brain-injured boy! It also made it possible for me to include my own observations, as well those of many family members who had a role in Caleb's story.

While the story was unfolding, Bettina and Bruce could scarcely keep up with the requests for news and updates. When their lives began to return to something like normal, in about February 2023, the story still demanded to be told.

Bettina's mother, Renate Kurschner, sensed there would be a great deal of interest in the saga, and remarked that it should become a book.

I agreed it would be a gripping story: the outcome was not at all a fore-gone conclusion, to a casual observer. Caleb's progress was unexpectedly swift, dramatic, and awe-inspiring, even to a non-religious person. In the case of most of Bruce and Bettina's family and community, their immediate response was to give thanks to God.

The process of putting the story together began with Renate Kur-schner and Bettina telling Caleb's story to a church event in Saskatch-ewan. Bettina assembled photographs on a projection screen. The photos, mostly taken by Bettina and Bruce, have been selectively used in this book, taking care to respect the privacy rights of those who are too young to give informed consent. How complicated life has become!

In addition to the photos, Bettina and Bruce maintained two records of Caleb's ordeal that were enormously helpful to me, once I took on the challenge of making this book happen. One was the lined notebook recording every medical treatment, every chart note, and every professional or family visitor for the first few days, then continu-ing as a diary. In this book, I found notes of what Caleb consumed, once he began eating. It was a ready-made logbook of the journey back from Middle Earth.

The second record-keeping exercise was the daily text messages to friends and relatives. About ninety percent of those messages are repro-duced in the pages of this book, with just a few of Bettina's exclamation marks. I left in enough so that her voice, not mine, is heard.

Bruce and Bettina were also able to obtain a copy of Caleb's medi-cal chart notes and test results, to take with them to Bloorview. This additional resource was a great help when exact medical terms were needed.

Caleb himself helped me to photocopy his medical file when he and Bruce came to our house for lunch on Sunday January 15, 2023. This was while he was still a patient at McMaster and was still seeing double. He was also happy to be interviewed by phone from Stewart Valley, a few weeks later. That was when he told me his analysis of "the dream," the part that I have designated as Middle Earth: he described being neither fully awake nor unconscious, but some other state of being.

Caleb and Eliza have known Jim and me since they were very young, but only for brief visits once or twice each year. In January 2023 we were able to spend some time with Eliza, in addition to the time Jim and I each spent in Caleb's hospital room. These opportunities to chat about normal things, like pets, favourite foods and school buses, made it easier for both children to feel comfortable with the idea that they would be in a book that I would write. Eliza was eager to tell me what she remembered about the night of Caleb's accident, and about how it was still troubling to her months later.

Once the narrative had a beginning, a middle and an ending, facts and details were filled in through interviews and many emails with Bettina and Bruce, and interviews with Dawn Pate, Brooke Newsome, Caleb Pate, Eliza Pate, Heather Pate and Doreen Pate.

ACKNOWLEDGEMENTS

The next step in the project, as with any manuscript, was to find beta readers, preferably readers who did not know the Pate family at all. Their job was to confirm what I was unable to judge: was the story as gripping and exciting as it seemed, or was I too close to the subjects?

For their remarks and helpful comments, corrections and patience, I would like to thank beta readers Donna Peters-Small, Dr. Dave Davis and Rev. Harold Munn. I am also indebted to Bettina Pate for endlessly correcting my mistakes, Jim Cairney for proof-reading and editorial advice, and Akosua Brown for all sorts of advice. I don't follow all the advice I get. Perhaps this is a character flaw. But thanks anyway.

ABOUT THE AUTHOR

Ann McRae is a writer and retired lawyer living in Dundas, Ontario. She and her husband Jim Cairney, a minister in the United Church of Canada, felt privileged to be part of Caleb Pate's story. Ann and Jim have two adult sons, three grandchildren and a dog.

Her first book, *Life, Love Loss and Other Four-Letter Words: Messages to Kathie* was published in 2020. It was followed by *Alia's Voice: A Syrian Refugee in Canada*, in 2022 (Kipekee Press). She is working on a children's book about a Syrian refugee, *Mousa from Nowhere*. She is also working on two biographies and a junior historical fiction series. As time permits, Ann is also a social justice activist and volunteer, a family historian, and a musician

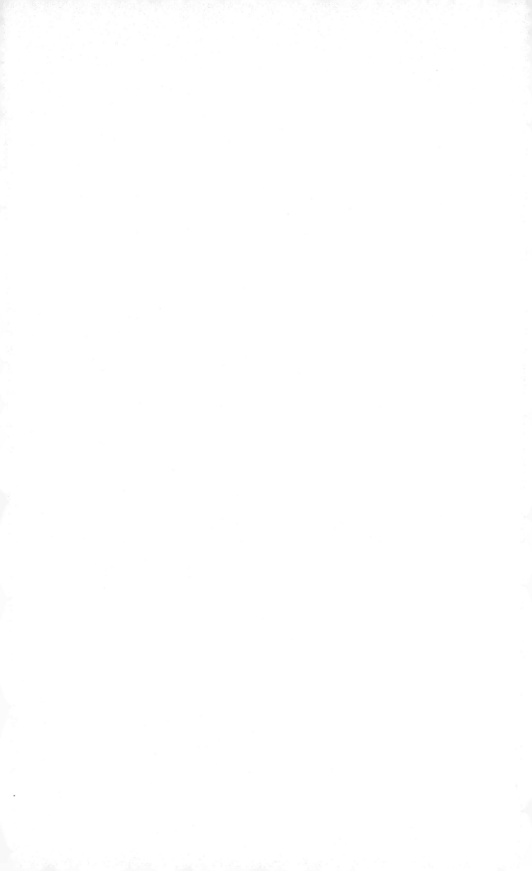

Made in United States
North Haven, CT
24 March 2025

67134588R00124